The Healthy House Answer Book

Published by:
The Healthy House Institute
430 North Sewell Road
Bloomington, IN 47408

Copyright © 1997 by John Bower and Lynn Marie Bower

Book and cover design by Lynn Marie Bower

Printed on recycled paper with soy-based ink.

10 9 8 7 6 5 4 3 2 1

Publisher's Cataloging-in-Publication Data.
Bower, John
      The Healthy House Answer Book: Answers to the 133
      most commonly asked questions / John Bower and
      Lynn Marie Bower
1. Housing and health. 2. Indoor air pollution—Health aspects.
3. Consumer education. I. Bower, Lynn Marie, joint author. II.
Title.

RA770.5.B69 1997
613'.5--dc 19

Library of Congress Catalog Card Number: 97-94365
ISBN 0-9637156-4-X $8.95 Softcover.

The Healthy House Answer Book

Answers to the 133 most commonly asked questions

by
John Bower
and
Lynn Marie Bower

The Healthy House Institute

Also by the authors

The Healthy House: How to buy one, how to build one, how to cure a sick one, by John Bower

The Healthy Household: A complete guide for creating a healthy indoor environment, by Lynn Marie Bower

Understanding Ventilation: How to design, select, and install residential ventilation systems, by John Bower

Healthy House Building: A design and construction guide, by John Bower

Your House, Your Health: A non-toxic building guide (VHS video), by John Bower and Lynn Marie Bower

Disclaimer

The information contained in this book should not be considered medical advice. Sensitive individuals should always contact a physician first before making any changes in their home environment.

Table of Contents

Preface

A healthy house is one that doesn't make you sick. While much has been written about the health of Mother Earth and environmental consciousness in general, the environment that's most likely to affect human health is inside our own homes. In fact, the indoor environment is actually responsible for a wide range of illnesses. Symptoms such as common allergies, fuzzy thinking, joint pain, anxiety, and death can all be caused by an unhealthy house.

We first became involved with healthy-house construction, and healthy life-styles, in 1984. Since that time, we've written about three-quarters-of-a-million words in several books and scores of articles describing healthy ways to build, decorate, and maintain houses. For a number of years, we offered a consulting service to answer specific questions from people. Because the questions were often very similar, and because we no longer have the time to offer personal consultations, we felt this book would be a great help to many people. It contains the 133 most commonly asked questions we've received over the years and, more importantly, the answers.

Introduction

If we would've been asked us in 1976 when we bought our first house if indoor pollution was an important issue, we probably would have said, "No." But we would have been wrong. A government report has stated that "Indoor air pollution...accounts for 50% of all illness (and) health care costs (from its effects) are estimated at $100 billion per year." That's an astounding statement. Think about all the times you, a friend, or a family member have been sick. Half of all those illnesses were probably caused by poor indoor air quality.

What we're talking about includes all forms of illness. Perhaps that case of the sniffles was due to a dust-mite allergy, or when you thought you had the flu, it was because of a malfunctioning chimney. Your grandfather's lung cancer may have been due to radon gas, and your daughter's menstrual irregularities could have been caused by the formaldehyde given off by the kitchen cabinets.

Many people have heard of Sick Building Syndrome. From time to time, the news media reports on a new office building where some employees are mysteriously ill. These people are healthy when they're away from work, but as soon as they get back on the job, they experience a variety of symptoms. Well, guess what? Houses can be sick, too.

We all have different levels of tolerance. In a sick office building, the air might only be bad enough to affect 10% of the workers. Similarly, houses usually aren't so bad that everyone gets seriously ill. In fact, in a typical sick house there's usually only one person affected. It's common for other family members, who feel OK, to label the sick person a hypochondriac.

One of the illnesses that's increasingly being recognized is a condition called Multiple Chemical Sensitivity (MCS). People with MCS are much more sensitive than the rest of the population to common indoor air pollutants. As with all illnesses, there are degrees of MCS. Some reports have estimated that it affects up to 15% of the population. We learned about MCS the hard way a few years after we bought out first house.

That house wasn't much to look at. It was a dilapidated Federal farm house that was built in the 1850s. Between 1976 and 1982, we completely rebuilt much of the inside and outside ourselves— while we were living in it. We were proud of the end result and where honored with a preservation award from the county historical society. But the exposure to all the new construction materials literally destroyed Lynn's health. It took us another couple of years to learn that many common building products can make you sick. Frankly, we were shocked. We had used the same plywood, cabinets, paints, and carpeting that anyone could buy at lumber yards and building-supply centers—and they almost destroyed Lynn.

At first we couldn't figure out why she has so many different and unrelated symptoms. She couldn't sleep and had joint and muscle pain. She couldn't digest food, couldn't think straight, and had inflamed sinuses. Her hair and nails became brittle. She had difficulty breathing, and the odor of printing ink and new clothing bothered her. Then we heard about MCS and realized that our award-winning house had made her sick. We found out that many doctors had never heard of MCS. While others had heard of it, they simply didn't believe it was a valid medical condition. But, we also learned there were several hundred doctors who specialized in treating MCS who saw thousands of patients every day. For a referral, contact the American Academy of Environmental Medicine (10 E. Randolph St., New Hope, PA 18938, 215-862-4544) or the American Academy of Otolaryngologic Allergists (8455 Colesville Rd., #745, Silver Springs, MD 20910, 301-588-1800).

Since becoming aware how bad the air is in most houses, as well as MCS, we've devoted out our lives to spreading the word about why houses make people sick and, more importantly, how to create healthy houses. We've found that even though many everyday materials are unhealthy, other products exist that are safer, better choices. This book discusses those healthy alternatives and includes addresses for some that you may have difficulty finding locally. Many of our answers include numbers in parentheses that refer to other questions and answers containing additional relevant information.

We've found that every question has two answers—a short one, and a long one. For example, it's possible to answer a particular question with either a single sentence, or an entire book. What follows are relatively short answers. However, they're certainly not incomplete. By following the advice given in these pages, you can definitely improve the healthfulness of your house and your family—often considerably.

Even if you're after more in-depth information, this is an excellent book with which to start because it will give you an overall background in all aspects of healthy housing.

John and Lynn Marie Bower
The Healthy House Institute

I.
Why are houses unhealthy?

I.

1. Have houses always been unhealthy or this something new?

Over the centuries, many houses have been unhealthy due to mold, wood smoke, gas lighting, kerosene heaters, coal dust, pests, animal dander, lead pipes, lead paint, asbestos, etc. While some of these pollutants are less common today, we now have new pollutants such as formaldehyde with which to contend. So, although unhealthy houses have been around for a while, the specific pollutants are changing.

2. With all the new environmental laws and regulations, why aren't houses healthier than ever before?

In some areas, there definitely has been some progress. For example, we no longer use lead paint or asbestos insulation. But in many instances, we're creating new building products and developing new construction practices faster than they can be evaluated or regulated. Today's indoor environmental pollution problems are related to two trends—the use of unhealthy *materials* and unhealthy *techniques*.

3. What are the two trends that are contributing to make today's houses unhealthy?

First of all, we're now building houses tighter for greater energy efficiency, but without mechanical ventilation systems. And second, we're filling these tighter houses with synthetic, man-made building materials, furnishings, and cleaning products—many of which release pollutants into the air. So, we end up with pollution-filled houses that don't have enough fresh air. The result is often ill health.

4. How bad is the air in a typical home?

According to many studies, the air inside most houses is 5 to 10 times worse than the outdoor air. And it doesn't matter where you live—in a major city, or in a rural area—the air is almost always worse indoors. If you measure individual pollutants, some are a whopping 100 times worse indoors.

5. What are the types of contaminants that are often found indoors?

We usually put them into six categories:
•*Biologicals* (pollutants that are, or once were, alive) such as mold, mildew, pollen, dust mites, animal dander, bacteria, and viruses.

- *Gases* resulting from human and pet metabolism (ammonia, certain alcohols, carbon dioxide, methane, etc.), gases that are by-products of combustion (carbon dioxide, carbon monoxide, sulfur dioxide, etc.), and gases that are released by synthetic and man-made products (formaldehyde, hexane, toluene, etc.).
- *Metals* such as lead (which used to be popular in paint), mercury (once used as a fungicide in paint and drywall compound), arsenic and chromium (widely used in chemically treated lumber).
- *Minerals* such as asbestos (found in some older insulation, vinyl tiles, and drywall compounds), mineral fibers and particles from fiberglass insulation, and air-borne minerals spewed out of humidifiers from tap water.
- *Radiation* from naturally occurring radon, electromagnetic radiation from wiring and electrical appliances, and radioactive waste in some smoke detectors and compact-fluorescent lamps. ⟶to
- *Vapors,* which in most houses means too much water vapor, something that can lead pollutant problems such as mold growth—or rot.

6. What are VOCs and could they be big polluters in my home?

VOC stands for *volatile organic compound.* There are hundreds of different VOCs and they have two things in common—they contain carbon, and they evaporate quickly. Some are natural and relatively benign—baking bread and cutting onions releases VOCs. But other VOCs are synthetic and aren't so safe to be around. They can be released by paints, solvents, caulking, and adhesives. Formaldehyde is probably the most recognized VOC. It's widely used in plywood, particle board, finishes, and many other products. Some VOCs are irritants, carcinogens, and mutagens. They can be serious indoor polluters.

7. What is outgassing?

Outgassing refers to release of VOCs as a material ages or degrades. New-car smell is composed of various gases that are released from the synthetic materials making up a new automobile's interior. As it turns out, many common building materials (carpeting, cabinets, paneling, paints, etc.) outgas harmful VOCs.

8. I'm fairly certain my house is making me sick. Should I hire a company to test the indoor air?

If you feel better when you're away from home, then get sick when you return, your house could indeed be making you sick. In some cases, professional air-quality testing can be helpful to understand why. But there are hundreds of possible pollutants, and testing for then all can cost hundreds, or thousands, of dollars. If you do such testing, you'll probably be given a list of perhaps a hundred pollutants unique to your house. Because there are so many pollutants that haven't been studied, you'll know what you've got, but you won't know what it means.

For the pollutants that have been studied, the guidelines as to what constitutes a safe exposure were often established for healthy workers in occupational settings. If you're hypersensitive, you could easily be bothered by much lower levels—levels many experts consider safe.

A little detective work on your part will often provide more useful information than air-quality testing. For example, ask yourself when your symptoms started. If it was after some remodeling, you should suspect the building materials. If it was after a new furnace was installed, your problem could be related to a fuel leak, combustion by-products, leaky ducts, or the materials the ducts are made of. If your house was recently weatherized, it may have been tightened to the point it no longer has enough fresh air, or the indoor air could have been contaminated with insulation. If you've had a flood, you should suspect mold. If you just built a new house, there can be a number of possibilities—outgassing from new materials, lack of ventilation, heating/cooling system problems, etc.

9. I've heard of something called a bakeout. Won't that increase the outgassing rate and get rid of the VOCs in my house?

A *bakeout* seems like the perfect solution. It involves heating a building up to about 95°F for three days or so, while simultaneously airing it out with window fans. This is a simple solution to a complex problem, and it doesn't always help. In fact, some studies have shown that the levels of some pollutants can actually increase after a bakeout.

10. How long does it take for a typical house to air out on its own?

This is a difficult question to answer because there are so many variables. For example, different brands of similar products outgas at different rates, the rate changes at different temperatures and humidities, and natural (or mechanical) ventilation is a factor. Plus each different VOC has it's own particular outgassing characteristics. As an example, formaldehyde (which is commonly used in kitchen cabinets and wall paneling) typically has a half-life of 3 to 5 years. So, these products will only lose half their formaldehyde in that time. And it'll take another 3 to 5 years for half of the remaining formaldehyde to be released, and so on. Because outgassing decreases with time, older houses often have lower levels of VOCs than new houses—if they've been maintained with healthy cleaning products and there's been no recent remodeling.

II.
The basics of healthy house construction

II.

11. Are there any particular products that stand out as being serious indoor polluters?

Yes, we call them *The Big Three.* They include *manufactured wood products,* which give off a lot of formaldehyde such as particle board and furniture-grade plywood. These materials are almost universally used in paneling and cabinetry.

Carpeting is a problem because it harbors vast quantities of dirt, dust mites, and other allergy-provoking particles. Carpet fibers, padding, chemical treatments, and cleaning products can also outgas dozens of harmful chemicals (#99).

Combustion appliances can be bothersome—if they aren't totally sealed. This includes such things as wood stoves, fireplaces, gas ranges, and many gas and oil hot water heaters and furnaces. They're dangerous because they can inadvertently introduce noxious gases such as carbon monoxide into the air you breathe (#65).

Eliminating these items will help to create what we call a *generically* healthy house—one that is considerably healthier than most homes. However, it may not healthy enough for people who are more sensitive than average, or for people who want the best possible indoor air quality.

12. Do you have a particular set of guidelines you follow?

We advocate three *Healthy-House Design Principles.* These are *Eliminate* pollutant sources by using healthier alternatives wherever possible, *Separate* from the living space any polluting materials you can't completely eliminate, and *Ventilate* to remove stale, polluted air and bring in fresh air. Sometimes *filtration* is listed as a fourth design point, but it's often combined with ventilation.

13. Won't building a house out of adobe, rammed earth, or straw bales create a naturally healthy house by eliminating synthetic and man-made products?

It's possible to build *any* type of home in a healthy manner. But, just because a house is constructed of natural materials doesn't necessarily mean it's healthy. After all lead, radon, and asbestos are natural. Plus, houses that have poor ventilation, improper water drainage, or high indoor humidity can be very unhealthy—no matter what materials are used.

Our focus is on creating homes with healthy indoor air. Some of the most benign materials are natural, but others are man-made. So, whether you prefer back-to-nature or high-tech, you should still choose products carefully.

14. What if I'm chemically sensitive? How careful do I need to be?

The design and construction of your house should follow the three Healthy-House Design Principles closely with an emphasis on eliminating as many potentially bothersome materials within the living space as feasible. Because everyone's tolerance level and metabolism is different, you should test any questionable materials for personal tolerance. (#15) While this book will cover the basics, you'll probably want to get some more detained information about healthy construction. We heartily recommend two of John's other books, *The Healthy House* and *Healthy House Building,* both of which contain a wealth of in-depth information.

15. How do I perform tolerability testing?

If you're very chemically sensitive, you should only do tolerability testing under your physician's supervision. For people who are only moderately sensitive, an overnight bedside test can often be helpful. Here's how we test paint.

Because all paints have an odor when wet, have someone else coat one side of a piece of aluminum foil (2-3' long) with a paint you believe you might tolerate. Write down the date and the brand, then set the sample aside in a little-used, well-ventilated room (or in an uncontaminated garage) until it seems to have lost its odor. Then lightly sniff the sample. If you detect any odor, set the sample

aside for another week. When you can't smell anything, place the sample next to your bed on the night
stand near your head. If you sleep well through the
night, the product is probably going to be tolerable.
Keep in mind, that a small sample is not going to be
as potent as a large wall. So, while this test is certainly not perfect, it's often a very useful tolerability
indicator.

16. How much does a healthy house cost?

There's no precise figure as to how much a
healthy house costs. It depends on the degree of
healthfulness (generically healthy or
hypoallergenically healthy), the size (small houses
are less costly that large ones), land values, labor
costs, and the luxuriousness of the materials (marble
floors vs. colored concrete). There's really a considerable range in costs. Some people have built healthy
houses for almost the same amount of money as
unhealthy houses, but others have spent as much as
25% more than for a typical house.

17. I want a healthy house but I just don't know if I can really afford one. What do you suggest?

We believe in *downsizing*, That is, building a
slightly smaller home. That way, you can put your
money into healthy materials and a good ventilation
system rather than extra little-used square footage. If

money is particularly tight, don't worry about the materials used outdoors such as roofing and siding. Concentrate on the materials actually inside the living space.

Here's something else to consider. If you build an unhealthy house, you may be spending extra money anyway—at the doctor's office. In choosing between the lesser of two evils, where would you rather have your money go—to a mortgage payment or toward medical expenses?

18. How do I find a designer or architect that can design a healthy house?

Currently, there's no national listing of healthy designers or architects. If you can't find someone who understands healthy design, those who specialize in solar or energy-efficient projects are often receptive. Whoever you choose, he or she should be someone with whom you feel comfortable. We highly recommend giving your designer or architect some healthy-house books to familiarize them with the concepts.

19. How do I find a contractor to build a healthy house?

There isn't any listing of healthy-house builders either. We've found that custom builders, or those who enjoy remodeling work, are often receptive because they're used to doing things differently on each project. Builders who specialize in energy-efficient construction are also good because they usually build to careful standards and are familiar with mechanical ventilation. Check with the Energy Efficient Building Association (2950 Metro Dr. #108, Minneapolis, MN 55425, 612-851-9940) to see if they have any members in your area. Again, whoever you choose, make sure they have copies of your healthy-house books.

Once your healthy house is under construction, it's a good idea to place a sign in a conspicuous spot on the site that reads, "This home is being specially built to insure pristine indoor air quality. Therefore, do not smoke in or around the house, or use any product that hasn't been specifically approved. Your understanding is much appreciated. Thank you." You might hold a preconstruction meeting for everyone involved to explain the scope of the project. The more knowledge workers have, the better job they will do, and the healthier your house will be.

20. We're in the middle of the construction process and my builder wants to use some unhealthy materials. What should I do?

You're the one paying the bills, so you're the boss. You have two choices: You can stick to your guns and tell him to use healthy materials, or cave in and let him build you an unhealthy house. In most cases, you should be able to work out a compromise.

But in some instances, homeowners have found it necessary to fire their builder and have someone else complete the job. Of course, this can get into a legal and financial mess. The best thing is to have a detailed set of plans in the first place with everything spelled out as to what materials are to be used and how changes are handled once construction begins.

21. What part of the country is the best place in which to build a healthy house?

There aren't many utopias anywhere in the world. However, virtually every state has some areas where the outdoor air is of reasonably good quality. When looking at a prospective building site, you'll want to consider a number of factors. For example, what's upwind of the area—chemically sprayed farm fields, busy highways, incinerators, smokestack industries, perhaps a sulfur-spewing volcano, etc.? Is the site on high or low land?

Higher land often has fewer drainage problems and better-quality air. Are there strong electromagnetic fields in the area from power substations, large transformers, or high-voltage power lines? How near are the neighbors, and what is their life-style? Do they routinely use wood stoves or lawn-chemical services? Does the site have an undesirable past? Perhaps it was a local landfill. Is the area known for extremely high radon readings? Is there any vegetation on the site that could be a problem—odorous creosote bushes, cedar trees, or pollen-bearing plants?

III.
Foundations, decks, and garages

III.

22. What do you think is the healthiest type of foundation?

There are four basic foundation types: concrete slab, crawl space, basement, and pier. In general, pier foundations are the easiest to build in a healthy manner because they lift a house up off the ground. When a house is well separated from the soil, it's more difficult for radon, subterranean termites, and ground moisture to get into the living space. Pier foundations are often used on hillside lots or in hot/humid climates.

Actually, we feel that any foundation can be healthy—if constructed and maintained carefully. You need to be concerned with moisture (both liquid water and relative humidity) which can lead to mold or rot, radon (a cause of lung cancer), subterranean-termite control (toxic chemicals should be avoided whenever possible), energy savings (to minimize heating/cooling expenses, and reduce the potential for condensation), and selecting materials that are inherently healthy.

23. Don't concrete slab foundations tend to be damp and moldy?

No, not if they're constructed correctly. We've built healthy concrete slabs several times and like them because they can easily be surfaced with a covering of low-tox ceramic tile. If you're on a very tight budget, a colored concrete slab decorated with natural-fiber area rugs can be an attractive choice. And, it can still be covered with tile later, when you have some extra cash.

Actually, we've found that very few sensitive people react to concrete. This is especially true if no chemicals (usually called *admixtures)* are used in the basic concrete mix. You should also avoid chemical curing compounds—misting water on a slab will keep it moist so it will cure slowly and naturally.

24. I want to use concrete foundation walls for a basement or crawl space. Is there a healthy form-release agent and dampproofing material?

Contractors usually coat wood or metal foundation forms with a petroleum-based oil so they won't stick to the concrete. However, the oil often contaminates the concrete enough to bother sensitive people. Although it costs a little more, some people have had very good luck by simply using a vegetable cooking oil instead. But if the forms are already saturated with petroleum-based oil from past jobs, a better solution is to first line them with polyethylene plastic sheeting. That way, after they've been filled with concrete, which has then cured, and the forms removed, the plastic can be easily peeled off.

Dampproofing coatings are often black, odorous, tar-like compounds. Because they're on the outside of the foundation wall, they aren't directly exposed to the living space, so they usually don't often affect the indoor air quality. But in rare instances, they can, so sensitive people often substitute a dampproofing made with Portland-cement—just to be safe. Thoroseal is one popular brand, but there are others.

25. We're considering a new house with either a crawl space or basement. Which is healthier?

That's a little like comparing apples and oranges. In new construction, both must address the issues of radon, moisture, materials, and termites—but they usually do so in different ways. If care is taken in design and construction, either can be a good choice.

A basement is healthiest—if it's considered living space. It should be conditioned, ventilated, filtered, and not be shut off from the rest of the house. This will help keep the basement air fresh. While there are certainly basements that are built incorrectly (#52), the rules for constructing basements properly are fairly straightforward and understood by many builders. The rules for building crawl spaces, on the other hand, can be in conflict with each other—depending on the season.

Crawl spaces usually have vents around their perimeters. When the vents are closed, a crawl space is somewhat like indoor space. For example, it's warmer than the outdoors in the winter, so water pipes won't freeze. But when the vents are open, there's more of an exchange of air with the outdoors, so it's more like outdoor space than indoor space. In reality, most crawl spaces are neither indoor nor outdoor spaces, they behave differently in summer than in winter, and they often have moisture problems. There are two solutions. Some experts advocate either building a crawl space like a short, tightly constructed, insulated basement *without vents* (this may be in violation of some building codes) and treating it like living space year round. Others suggest leaving all the vents open and treating it like outdoor space all year. (Be sure to insulate those water pipes!).

If you have an existing basement or crawl space that's contaminated with moisture, mold, radon, or termite chemicals, you'll first need to do some remedial work by using the Healthy-House Design Principles of eliminate, separate, and ventilate (#12). It's imperative that you carefully analyze why the basement or crawl space is contaminated before you try to fix it. Otherwise, you can spend a great deal of money and not solve the problem. Because some situations are difficult to diagnose, you may want to consult an expert for some advice. We've found that companies that do pre-purchase home inspections are often very helpful.

26. Do think it's worth the expense of installing a radon mitigation system in a new house?

Radon mitigation means taking measures to minimize radon levels indoors. That's a good idea because radon causes cancer, so it's a pollutant that should be treated with respect. But, the only way to tell if the radon level is too high is to actually measure the concentration of radon in the indoor air—and you can't do that until the house is completed.

To answer the question, we're going to rephrase it a little: "Should we install a radon mitigation system as the house is being built, or should we wait until the house is completed, then measure the radon level indoors and determine if we need a system at that time?"

Because most radon comes from the soil, what we think seems to make the most sense is to design the foundation to prevent radon from entering the house. And, as the house is being built, install part of a mitigation system. Don't install the whole ball-of-wax, just put in enough to make it easy to hook up the rest of a system later—if you need it. After the house is finished, if you find radon mitigation is necessary, it's easy and relatively inexpensive to install. If you don't need radon mitigation, you really haven't spent much extra money. This is just like buying insurance.

If you're building a basement, for example, you might install some inexpensive perforated plastic pipe under the basement floor slab and connect it to a capped tee fitting that sticks up through the floor. Then after the house is finished, you can measure the radon concentration in the basement. (You can buy radon test kits at many hardware stores.) If the concentration is too high, you simply hook up an exhaust fan to the tee and connect the fan to the outdoors with another length of pipe. This will pull the radon from under the slab (before it has a chance to enter the basement) and blow it outside into the atmosphere. If you measure a low radon level in the basement, you don't need to do anything further. You can get more information about radon testing and mitigation from the EPA's indoor-air-quality infoline at 800-438-4318.

27. I'm very concerned about having toxic chemicals around my home's foundation. How do I safely deal with termites?

There are several types of termites in the U.S., but the most common, and most destructive, is the subterranean termite. They live in nests in the soil, and continually travel back and forth from their nest to the wooden parts of a house. If they're exposed to the air for very long, their bodies dry out quickly and they die. So, they often travel inside hollow concrete blocks, or they build mud tubes to move through.

For decades, toxic chemicals called termiticides (termite killers) have been routinely used around foundations either as a preventive measure or to halt an existing termite infestation. Now, fortunately, there are some less noxious control methods available.

There are actually several less-toxic alternatives, some of which look promising. For example, Dow Elanco (9330 Zionsville Rd., Indianapolis, IN, 46268, 800-352-6776) has developed a Sentricon system that involves placing underground bait stations around a house to attract termites. The bait contains a low-tox chemical that prevents termites from molting. As a result, after they eat it, they eventually die. This can be used with either new or existing houses.

U.S. Borax (26877 Tourney Rd., Valencia, CA 91355, 800-984-6267) has a low-tox chemical called Tim-Bor which can be sprayed on wood to permanently poison it so termites won't eat it. While Tim-Bor shouldn't be ingested, it's basically a mineral, so it doesn't release any odors or gases into the air. It's big drawback is the fact that it remains water soluble, so it can't be exposed to rain. In new construction, you wait until the house is under roof and is closed in, then you can walk around the inside and spray a Tim-Bor/water solution on all the wood in the house. In an existing house, you can certainly spray any exposed wood in a basement or crawl space, but there will usually be some parts of a house that are hidden and can't be sprayed.

Another solution for new construction is called a *sand-barrier.* It involves placing a layer of sand around the perimeter of the foundation. The sand *must* be a certain grain size—the particles must be too big and heavy for the termites to move out of the way to tunnel through, yet too small for them to fit between the grains. Termites will go to great lengths to find wood to eat. Therefore, sand barriers must be placed carefully to avoid pathways around the sand.

Termite shields are made of galvanized steel or aluminum and they're placed on top of the foundation to block the termites on their way to the upper wooden parts of a house. However, shields often aren't totally effective because the termites can build their mud tubes around the shields and get to the wood portions of a house anyway. What the shields do is force the termites out into the open, so you'll be able to see their mud tubes early—before any structural damage is done.

One of the best sources for information about alternative or less-toxic control of termites (or any pest for that matter) is the Bio-Integral Resource Center (P.O. Box 7414, Berkeley CA 94707, 510-524-2567).

28. My contractor wants to use salt-treated lumber for my outdoor deck. Is there anything unhealthy about it?

Most of this lumber is pine that's been pressure treated with toxic copper, chromium, and arsenic salts—not table salt. Sometimes there's a white arsenic powder on the wood. Manufacturers warn that you should wear gloves and respiratory and eye protection when working with it, and that you should wash your clothes separately from other laundry. Furthermore, treated wood should not be used for eating surfaces (picnic tables), and you should never burn the scraps.

Workers are at much more risk than homeowners because they can easily inhale the chemically laden sawdust. However, we're also concerned about children playing on treated decks and playground equipment.

The simplest solution is to use redwood instead of salt-treated lumber. It has little odor, so it's often tolerable to people who are bothered by the smell of pine, it's naturally resistant to insect attack, and it needs no sealer. It does cost more than treated lumber. But, construction-grade redwood (it has a few knots in it) isn't excessively expensive. As a reasonable compromise, you might use treated lumber for the support structure (the posts embedded in the ground and the floor joists), then use redwood for all the exposed surfaces (the deck itself and the railings).

Redwood ages to a natural gray color, but can eventually get quite dark. To clean it, we use a scrubber sponge and low-tox liquid detergent, then rinse.

29. I like the convenience of an attached garage, but aren't detached garages healthier?

Garages are routinely filled with exhaust gases and gasoline odors. A hot automobile can also smell of oil or rubber. Garages also often contain lawn chemicals, paints and solvents, insecticides, etc., all of which can leak into the living space through unseen gaps and cracks in the common walls or ceiling. Contaminants can also get into the indoor air if there are leaky heating/cooling ducts in the garage. It's not unusual for odors and combustion gases to rise up into bedrooms located above a garage.

The easiest way to prevent these pollutants from getting into the living space is to build a detached garage. This works best if the garage is downwind of the house. If you have your heart set on an attached garage, you should build it as airtight as possible (#37). In other words, every possible pathway between the garage and the living space should be sealed. This typically involves using gaskets in some places between the drywall and the framing, caulking or aerosol foam insulation, weather-stripping around the service door leading into the house, and airtight electrical boxes and light fixtures. But even if all this is done, some pollutants will enter whenever the service door is opened.

Something that can improve the air quality in all garages is an exhaust fan controlled by a spring-wound crank timer. After pulling a hot automobile (or motorcycle, or lawn mower) into the garage, you can crank the timer around for an hour or so. This will air out the garage while the vehicle cools down, then the timer will shut the fan off automatically. An exhaust fan can also help when you first start up an automobile in the morning, but its best to pull the car outdoors and let it warm up there.

IV.
Framing and insulation

IV.

30. We're considering building a house with steel framing. Does it have any particular advantages?

Light-weight steel framing is becoming popular with some builders. It consists of C-shaped studs and channels that are usually lighter-in-weight than wood. Everything is held together with self-tapping screws, and the studs typically have holes prepunched in them for electrical wires and plumbing lines. This saves drilling time, but the holes have sharp edges, so they must be fitted with plastic grommets to prevent plastic-jacketed wiring from getting nicked and shorting out. Steel framing is also very uniform in size, it has no knots, and it won't warp.

The biggest health-related advantage to steel is the fact that it never needs to be treated for termites. So, where toxic chemical use is the norm, or where less-toxic alternative treatments (#27) aren't feasible, steel is a great option.

Although it's not a concern for most people, some very sensitive individuals are bothered by the natural odor of wood, and steel is odor-free. Most framing lumber is pine or another softwood, and the odor is composed of the same chemicals in turpentine. These sensitive people are just reacting to much lower levels of the same pollutants that have the potential to bother all of us.

While steel itself usually doesn't have an odor, it sometimes has a slightly odorous oil film on it left over from the manufacturing process that some sensitive people have had to wash off. A solution of water and TSP (tri-sodium phosphate, a heavy-duty cleaner often available in hardware stores) usually works well.

31. Are there any disadvantages to using steel framing?

The biggest disadvantage to building with steel has to do with the fact that steel is an excellent conductor of heat. An insulated steel-framed wall can be very energy inefficient. For example, there can be so much heat loss through steel studs, that the *average* insulating ability of the wall is degraded by up to 50%. This can be a serious drawback—especially in harsh climates—but there are some ways to minimize energy losses. For example, you can space the studs further apart. Fewer studs equals less heat loss.

Most residential builders have never worked with steel, so they don't really understand some of the unique details that go into a steel-framed house. While the actual cost of the material is often comparable to wood framing, if a contractor is unfamiliar with steel, he may charge more for labor.

There are a few specialized tools required—a screw gun, a cut-off saw fitted with a steel-cutting blade, some tin snips, and perhaps a crimping tool.

Plus, you'll need a selection of self-tapping screws—they come in dozens of sizes and shapes.

32. Does it matter what kind of sheathing we use on our house?

There are negative health affects related to most sheathing materials. For example, there are several different kinds of foam boards that are relatively odorless. However, some release chemicals that can damage the Earth's protective ozone layer. In a fire, foam sheathing gives off very toxic gases. Asphalt-impregnated fiberboard sheathing has a slight asphalt odor. Gypsum-board sheathing has a facing paper that's chemically treated, and plywood and oriented-strand board contain formaldehyde-based glue.

The good news is that health effects related to sheathing usually aren't significant. One of the reasons is because materials outside the living space don't tend to have a serious affect on indoor air quality. Actually, the sheathing is inside the wall cavity—sandwiched between the siding and the interior wallboard—so it can't outgas inward or outward very easily.

Still, sheathing can bother some very sensitive people. For them, the solution may mean eliminating sheathing. This is possible, but you must analyze the situation carefully—and make sure you don't violate any building codes. If you build a house as airtight as possible (#37), the materials inside wall cavities are almost never a health problem.

33. Do you think housewrap is needed on my new house?

Housewrap is a plastic fabric-like material sold in wide rolls. It's designed to be stapled over the exterior sheathing of a home and act as a wind barrier. By preventing the wind from blowing through the cracks, it can improve the energy efficiency of a house. Most brands have little odor. And, as with sheathing, housewrap is always covered up with siding, so you're not exposed to it directly.

Some very sensitive people have used an aluminum-foil-faced Kraft paper, called builders foil or reflective insulation, as house wrap. Plastic housewrap is manufactured so, in cold climates, moisture will pass through it, rather than become trapped inside the wall cavity. So if you opt for builder's foil in a cold climate, you should get the type that has tiny pin pricks in it. This perforated product will still block the wind, but it won't trap water vapor. Mail-order suppliers of builders foil include E.L. Foust Co. (P.O. Box 105, Elmhurst, IL 60126, 800-225-9549) and Nontoxic Environments, Inc. (P.O. Box 384, New Market, NH 03857, 800-789-4348).

34. What does the term R-value refer to?

When you buy insulation, it will have an R-value such as R-13 or R-38. This is a measure of how well a material resists the flow of heat, so the higher the number, the better it's insulating ability. However, there's more to heat loss than R-value. For example, a house can have walls filled with plenty of insulation having a high R-valve, yet be costly to heat or cool. This is usually because the house is leaky, and there's a significant amount of air moving through those leaks. Leaking air can carry a great deal of conditioned air with it. So, making a house energy efficient takes a combination of R-value and tightening.

35. What options do I have for insulation?

The bad news is, there are negative health effects associated will all insulations. The good news is, in most cases, we've found insulation stays inside building cavities where it's been placed, and usually doesn't affect the indoor air quality. Of course, there are horror stories where insulation has been responsible for very serious health problems. Therefore, it pays to select and install it with care.

In the 1970s, a product called urea-formaldehyde foam insulation was in use that was capable of releasing a great deal of formaldehyde. It hasn't been around for some time, but there are a number of other foams on the market today. Some are sold primarily in 4' x 8' sheets, while others require special equipment to foam them in place inside walls, floors, and roofs. Once cured, there isn't a great deal of outgassing from any of these newer foams—but there is a little. And, many can give off toxic gases when they burn. As a result, most building codes require that they be covered with something such as drywall. Once covered up, they're never directly exposed to the living space.

Fiberglass is one of the most widely-used residential insulations. It can be unhealthy for two reasons. There is some evidence that tiny glass fibers, when they're inhaled, can lodge in the lungs and possibly result in lung cancer. In addition, most fiberglass insulation is held together with a formalde-hyde-based resin. The resin isn't a strong outgasser, but it can bother sensitive people.

Cellulose insulation is made from ground-up newspapers. It's very dusty and can be contaminated with printing ink, mold, and flame-retardant chemicals. Cellulose is often installed in existing walls by blowing (injecting) it under pressure through small holes drilled in the siding (or through the interior wallboard). When this is done, a certain amount of insulation can be blown into the living space. (Chopped fiberglass can also be installed in this way.) In new construction, cellulose insulation is sometimes mixed with a tiny amount of glue or water and sprayed into wall cavities before they're covered with drywall. In all applications, once installed, the insulation is outside the living space.

Cotton insulation is now being made by Greenwood Cotton Insulation Products (P.O. Box 1017, Greenwood, SC 29648, 800-546-1332). It's billed as being more environmentally responsible because it's made from recycled cotton jeans—and cotton is a renewable crop. However, it isn't perfect. It must be hand-fluffed to reach its full thickness. And it isn't 100%-cotton_it contains some polyester and is treated with a boric-acid flame retardant.

There are other materials that can be used for insulation, such as cork, feathers, straw, etc. All have advantages and disadvantages. The perfect insulation simply doesn't exist.

36. So, what's the healthiest insulation to use in my house?

This is one of our most often asked questions. While the residential insulations in common use all have drawbacks, they've all been used in healthy construction. In fact, wherever there have been serious health problems associated with insulation, it's usually resulted from exposures during installation or remodeling when the insulation is being disturbed. It's been our experience that if you're concerned about your health, it's much more important how the insulation is installed, than which product is used.

If you have an existing house and you want to add some insulation, it should be done with care. This is because, the installation process itself often contaminates the interior of the house. This is particularly true if cellulose or fiberglass is blown into building cavities. In most cases, there will be bits of fiberglass or cellulose floating around indoors, and perhaps small piles of insulation on the floor near electrical receptacles or light switches. In some cases, heating ducts have been inadvertently filled with insulation, or insulation has been sucked into leaky ducts (#69). We recommend, during the actual insulating process, a workman be indoors to make sure there are no significant amounts of insulation filtering into the living space. Then, after the job is finished, the interior should be cleaned up thoroughly. In most cases, the insulation will be packed fairly tightly inside the walls—and it will probably stay there. However, some could filter into the living space later, from the walls or attic. If this happens, you should determine where it's entering and caulk, or otherwise seal the pathways. (Be sure to check for leaky ducts.) Once that's been done, the insulation probably will no longer pose problems.

In new construction we recommend that the house be built as tightly as possible (#37). That way, whatever insulation you choose, it will be very well separated from the living space. If it can't get into the air you breathe, then it can't affect your health.

37. I thought tight houses caused indoor air pollution. Why are saying they're a good idea?

The people who claim that tight houses are a problem don't understand the whole picture. As far as indoor air quality is concerned, the unhealthiest houses are those built with polluting materials and having no mechanical ventilation. These houses often have a problem no matter how loose they are. However, the indoor air quality is worse, if they're tightly built. By the way, loose houses also have other disadvantages. They're often expensive to heat and cool, too dry in the winter, drafty, and uncomfortable (#76).

The healthiest houses are actually built as tight as possible—using both healthy materials and a mechanical ventilation system. This results in a number of advantages. For example, a tight house is more energy efficient, and quieter. It's less likely to develop hidden moisture problems inside building cavities. Pollutants in the soil (such as radon and termite chemicals) can't enter easily it. Pollutants inside the building cavities, such as insulation (or the slight odor of pine framing), can't enter easily it either. Because healthy materials were chosen, there aren't any significant pollution sources indoors causing problems. The mechanical ventilation system provides the correct amount of ventilation at all times—neither too much to be wasteful, nor too little. And, finally, if there is an outdoor pollution alert (say, a neighbor is spraying nasty chemicals on his fruit trees), the air coming in through the ventilation system can be filtered. The entire ventilation system can even be temporarily turned off. With loose construction you have no such control.

There are several techniques and materials that can be used to tighten a house. We've used gaskets, caulking, aerosol-foam insulation, and airtight electrical boxes. The goal is to seal all the many cracks and gaps that can be found between all the different building materials (#38). The Energy Efficient Building Association (2950 Metro Dr. #108, Minneapolis, MN 55425, 612-851-9940) offers books on tight construction techniques. John's *Healthy House Building* book shows how to build an airtight healthy house in a step-by-step manner.

38. What's a vapor barrier and should I use one?

A vapor barrier is more correctly called a diffusion retarder. That's because most materials aren't really perfect *barriers*, so *retarder* is a more accurate term. Plus, they tend to retard not only vapors but gases as well that are moving through materials by a process called *diffusion*.

There's often some confusion between airtight (#37) and diffusion-tight. In airtight construction, you seal up all the small holes and pathways that air can move through due to differing air-pressures. For example, when the wind blows on the side of a typical house, it pushes air, and airborne pollutants, through the cracks and gaps. But, with airtight construction, there aren't unplanned, cracks and gaps. As a result, the wind can't push any air or pollutants through to the interior living space.

On the other hand, diffusion-tight means greatly reducing the movement of gases and vapors (not particles) through a solid surface. The speed with which they pass through a material depends on their concentration in the air, and on the material's composition. Diffusion is faster through cardboard and drywall than through glass and metal.

If you study the laws of physics that apply, you'll see that in most houses, 100 times more air (with or without pollutants) is traveling through the tiny gaps and cracks than is moving by diffusion through all the solid surfaces combined! So, if you plug up the holes by making a house airtight, you've stopped 99% of the air and pollutant movement. As it turns out, in most cases, diffusion isn't very significant.

There are a variety of products that retard diffusion quite well. Plastic sheeting is widely used, but the asphalt-impregnated paper on fiberglass insulation also works well. Aluminum foil (#90), glass, glazed ceramic tile (#108), and some paints also function as diffusion retarders. While some of these materials are slightly better at retarding diffusion than others, the differences are small. And, because diffusion isn't an important way for pollutants or moisture to move through surfaces, in practice, all work acceptably. Diffusion retarders are a good idea, easy to install, and widely used. However, they generally aren't as important as sealing up the cracks.

39. I'm bothered by the odors of both pine framing lumber and fiberglass insulation. If I build an airtight house, can I use them inside the walls?

You sure can. If there's an airtight wall between you and the pine framing and the insulation, you should be just fine. In fact, Lynn's bothered those same materials, too, and we built our own house with them. Once everything was sealed, she could no longer smell them indoors.

The interior partition walls between rooms usually aren't insulated, and it generally doesn't make sense to make them airtight. Therefore, for pine-sensitive people, we like to use light-gauge steel studs for partition walls. (#30, #31) That way, there's no pine odor within the airtight envelope.

V.
Windows, siding, and roofing

V.

40. Aren't wood windows best from a health standpoint?

Wood windows are usually treated with water-repellent and fungicidal chemicals. So, while wood is a natural material, treated windows can certainly bother some sensitive people. Also, they're usually made of pine which can have a strong natural odor. Furthermore, wood windows require routine painting. However, wood windows usually aren't strong outgassing sources. Therefore, these concerns are only important for very sensitive people.

Vinyl windows are a less-expensive option. While they never need painting (a real plus), the vinyl itself can outgas a little—especially when new—which can be enough to bother some sensitive individuals.

Personally, we prefer aluminum-framed windows. Most are available prefinished in white or brown, and they require little maintenance. In cold climates, you should look for frames with thermal-breaks to minimize sweating. Aluminum windows generally have rubber or plastic seals that have a slight odor—but it usually isn't significant.

Multiple panes of glass are a good idea in harsh climates for energy efficiency. Low-E coatings and argon-filled windows rarely cause health problems, and we think they're important to conserve energy.

41. Is there a healthy window putty I can use?

In the past, window putty used to be made with linseed oil and other ingredients, but today vinyl compounds are more common. Either can be odorous when fresh, but because the putty is applied to the exterior of a window, it's outside the living space, so it's usually not a serious problem. The putty tends to be less bothersome after aging for a while, or after being painted. We aren't aware of one brand that's less odorous than others.

42. Are there any healthy caulkings and construction adhesives?

All caulkings and adhesives have an odor when wet, but once cured, they tend to outgas very little. The goal is to select a long-lasting product (so you won't have to reapply it very often), and one that will outgas most of its odor within a short period.

Most water-based latex caulks are good choices because they outgas less than other types of caulking. Personally, we've had good luck with 100%-silicone caulking for most outdoor applications. It's reasonably priced, durable, and very long lasting. It does have a strong odor when fresh, but once it's had about a week or so to air out, it's quite inert. Silicone's a little messy to work with because it can't be cleaned up with water, and while it can't be painted, it's usually available in some basic colors.

For a healthy construction adhesive, several companies now make water-based products, and some offer zero-solvent adhesives. While they're all odorous during application, they air out fairly well, and are almost always covered up, so they're rarely exposed directly to the living space.

43. Is it all right to use vinyl siding on my new healthy house?

Vinyl siding does outgas a small amount, especially when warmed by the sun. And, in a fire, it melts and burns very quickly producing toxic gases. On the plus side, vinyl's big advantages include low-cost, availability, durability, and the color goes all the way through so scratches aren't noticeable.

Because siding is outside the living space, it usually doesn't have a significant impact on indoor air quality. But, some sensitive people are bothered by warm vinyl siding on a hot summer day when they're next to it, or indoors when the windows are open. We like aluminum or steel siding because it usually has an inert baked-on finish. Brick is also a popular, low-outgassing, low-maintenance siding. The big drawback to wood siding is the fact that it requires regular painting or staining.

We've talked to many people on a tight budget, for whom brick, aluminum, or steel are simply too expensive. They often choose vinyl siding, then concentrate on spending any extra money indoors where it will do the most good. We think that can be a wise decision.

44. What healthy paints and clear finishes can I use on my home's exterior?

Some of the most long-lasting paints contained toxic lead. Fortunately, they're no longer on the market, having been replaced with oil-based and water-based products. In general, the water-based varieties are less toxic because they air out much faster, so we prefer them.

There are a number of healthier-than-average interior paints (#93) but, because outdoor paints must withstand much harsher conditions, conventional off-the-shelf paints are the only ones we feel should be used outdoors. Alternative paints simply won't hold up to the rain, temperature extremes, and sunlight.

Very sensitive people may want to test two or three different brands to see if any one is less bothersome. But, in general, as long as you choose a good-quality water-based product, exterior paints generally don't affect the indoor air quality very much once they're dry.

One of biggest enemies of an outdoor finish is the ultraviolet from sunlight. Clear wood finishes don't last very long outdoors (sometimes only a year or two) because the sunlight goes through the finish and damages the wood itself. Once the wood is damaged, the finish no longer adheres very well, and soon flakes off. Stains last a little longer (depending on how much pigment they contain), but they often need to be reapplied every few years. So, to avoid regular reapplications and reexposures to fresh materials, we prefer paints outdoors rather than stains and clear finishes.

For outdoor metalwork (doors, railings, etc.), you might consider automotive paints. They're available in a wide variety of colors and, if you go to a body shop that has the equipment to bake the paint on, you'll end up with a very durable and inert finish.

45. Can the foam insulation inside a steel entry door be a problem?

Usually not, because the steel outer skin tends to minimizes outgassing from the insulation inside it. Actually, we like insulated steel doors for other reasons, as well. For example, they're warp-resistant and long-lasting. They're also energy efficient. Many have magnetic weather-stripping (like a refrigerator), and an adjustable threshold, so they seal very well. Finally, when painted with a baked-on automotive paint (#44), they're inert and virtually maintenance free.

Wood doors, on the other hand, often don't seal well, and they require frequent repainting. Plus, most wood doors are chemically treated with water-repellents and fungicides—although this usually isn't a serious issue.

46. Aren't cedar shingles or shakes the logical healthy choice for roofing?

Roofing materials are not only outside the living space, but they're also way up on the roof. Therefore, they usually don't affect the quality of the indoor air. However, cedar shingles are actually one of the most bothersome roofing materials because cedar is so aromatic. We've heard of cases where sensitive people reroofed with cedar and the odor permeated their homes.

Fiberglass and asphalt shingles are, by far, the most common residential roofing material. They can have an asphalt odor, but it's rarely a problem indoors. About the only time we've heard of people being bothered is when there's an open dormer window overlooking a hot roof in the summer.

In most cases, roofing is chosen because of it's appearance, expected life, and cost—rather than healthfulness.

47. Why do you use metal roofs on the healthy houses you build?

Granted, roofing usually doesn't affect the air inside a house. But our own personal philosophy is to use materials that are as inert as possible wherever we can.

Most metal roofing is coated with an baked-on finish that's quite inert. We like to use sheet roofing that can be screwed down to 2x4s that are attached to the rafters every 24" (the 2x4s are called purlins). That way, we don't need a plywood roof deck or asphalt-impregnated felt paper for an underlayment. Plus, we like the appearance of sheet-metal roofing.

VI.
Plumbing and moisture

VI.

48. Should I use metal or plastic water pipes in my new house?

Plastic water mains are now widely used by utilities, and they're also common in many new houses. They tend to be easier and less expensive to install than an metal pipes. Many plastic pipes use both a toxic solvent-based cleaner and cement to fuse the pipe and fittings together. While these are very noxious, they're so volatile that they outgas quickly—usually within a few hours—if there's plenty of extra ventilation.

When water moves through new plastic plumbing lines, many sensitive people report a plastic-like taste. This occurs if contaminants are being released into the water, either from the pipe itself or from the cleaner or glue.

While you can't do much about what your water utility uses for underground water mains, we prefer to use copper for supply lines inside houses. In the past, lead-based solder was common. But today, Federal regulations forbid the use of lead in plumbing solders. Galvanized-steel piping is also relatively inert, but it's usually more expensive than copper.

Drain pipes are bigger in diameter, making copper drains expensive. Therefore, we often recommend using plastic for these. The plastic really doesn't outgas very much into the air. But to minimize outgassing, we buy the pipe and fittings early in the construction process and let them air out before they're installed. Then, when the cleaner and glue are used, we stay away for a while and provide extra ventilation until everything has aired out.

Because plastic drains are almost always inside wall or floor cavities, they're rarely exposed directly to the living space. That means, they usually aren't an outgassing problem. Still, just to be extra safe, we often recommend to sensitive people that plastic drains be wrapped with household aluminum foil before the wallboard is installed over them.

49. Do you believe all houses need a water filter?

That's a tough question to answer. The goal isn't to obtain pure H_2O, because pure H_2O can be tasteless, and it's very purity makes it *aggressive*. Aggressive water will dissolve and grab minerals from whatever it touches. If you drink aggressive water, it can actually pull minerals out of your body—minerals you need for good health. So, you don't want to purify water too much.

Before you think about filtering at all, you should determine how polluted your water is. If you're on a public water utility, it should be able to give you a water-quality analysis which will tell you what contaminants are in the water. If you're on a private water supply (well, cistern, or pond), you'll probably need to have your water tested by a private laboratory. Many different contaminants are possible, and testing for all of them can be expensive. So, you might ask someone at a nearby utility which contaminants are most likely in your geographic area. They can also usually recommend a testing lab.

Personally, we feel that the chlorine added by most utilities is one of the nastier chemicals routinely found in drinking water. However, it's easy to remove with a simple *taste and odor filter* that you can often buy at hardware and discount department stores. These filters contain activated carbon, and they can be placed on the main incoming water supply line (as a *whole-house* filter) to filter all the water in the house. Unfortunately, some kinds of bacteria can live and multiply in an activated-carbon filter. With public water supplies, most of the harmful bacteria will have been killed by the chlorine, so activated carbon usually works well. But, with private supplies that haven't been disinfected, activated carbon may not be good idea

Depending on what your water testing reveals, you may (or may not) opt for a reverse-osmosis filter or a distiller. These are more complex than a simple activated-carbon filter, and they're usually only practical as under-sink filters to purify water that's used for drinking and cooking. When you only filter water at one particular location, it's called a *point-of-use* filter.

50. What do the different kinds of water filters remove?

There are many companies offering filters today. Big corporations like Sears and Culligan sell them, as well as many mail-order catalogs. We've even seen some at K-Mart. There are only a few common strategies, but some models combine more than one filtering method in a single unit.

The simplest filter is a *sediment* filter. It's only designed to remove gritty particles and dirt. It can be a good choice if your water is cloudy or muddy looking. (However, make sure the cloudiness is not made up of biological life forms!)

The *activated carbon* filters mentioned above (#49) will not only remove chlorine but also many other dissolved gases and pesticides. Some units have a plastic housing, but others are made of stainless steel. The plastic housings often aren't a problem for sensitive people because the activated carbon removes plasticky odors and tastes from the water. Some manufacturers use *solid, compressed, activated carbon*, which is a bit more effective than *granular activated carbon*. Some filters are large enough that they only need the cartridge changed a few times a year. Others need to be replaced every month or two—depending on water quality and usage. You can also buy small filters that can be fitted onto an individual faucet or shower head.

KDF filters are a fairly recent development. They're able to remove chlorine. In addition, they're good at removing lead and deactivating hard-water minerals. Another plus is that KDF filters inhibit bacterial growth, so a KDF filter unit rarely becomes contaminated with microorganisms. Whole-house KDF filters and point-of-use models are manufactured by Global Environmental Technologies (P.O. Box 8839, Allentown, PA 18105-8839, 800-800-TERRA).

Reverse osmosis units use a special membrane through which water passes. They can remove dissolved minerals, particulates, and many biological contaminants. Most are point-of-use kitchen models that have a built-in storage tank—which mounts under the sink—and a special faucet at the sink. They require electricity to operate and they waste several gallons of water down the drain for each gallon of filtered water they produce. Their membranes are unable to remove chlorine or dissolved gases.

Water distillers boil water. Solid contaminants are left in the bottom of the boiler unit and the purified steam is separated and cooled (either by room temperature or a cooling device) to produce the filtered water. Water distillers are good at removing particulates and microbes. However, some volatile gases can evaporate with the steam. Distillers produce filtered water slowly, they use electricity, and they require an under-sink storage tank. Most are made of stainless steel, but glass units are also available.

Water quality can be quite a complicated subject, so you may want to have a professional help you select a system—or read up a little more on it. Lynn's book, *The Healthy Household*, goes into much more depth on contaminants, strategies, and equipment than is possible here.

51. What type of humidifier is healthiest?

A number of people believe having a humidifier is essential for a healthy house—especially in dry climates or where the indoor air in winter gets excessively dry. Actually, humidifiers often cause more problems than they solve. In reality, most people can usually adapt to a relative humidity of 20% or lower. If you experience dry or irritated eyes and mucous membranes, the air might be too dry. But, it's often a combination of dry air *and* irritation caused by airborne contaminants that's really causing the discomfort.

Air that's too dry in the winter is usually the result of a house being overventilated because it's too loosely constructed. On the other hand, tight houses in cold climates often have comfortable indoor humidities. If part of the problem is poor indoor air quality, you should first work on the three Healthy-House Design Principles discussed earlier (#12).

There are two big health problems with humidifiers. Most of them are routinely contaminated with mold, bacteria, and a variety of other microorganisms that can become airborne and affect allergic people. Many units also spew irritating minerals into the air that were dissolved in the water (unless distilled water is used in them). While the best solution is to tighten the house so it isn't overventilated, and to improve the indoor air quality, admittedly, using a humidifier is an easier approach.

After considering all the pros and cons of the various humidifier types, we feel there are a couple that are better-than-average. You might look for a *steam unit*. The high heat will disinfect the water. For whole-house applications, a number of companies make *flow-through humidifiers* that can be used in forced-air heating systems. The flow-through types have several internal absorbent plates that water runs over. When air blows past the plates, moisture is transferred into the airstream. They don't have a reservoir, so mold growth is minimized, but a certain amount of water is lost down the drain whenever they're operating.

Whatever type of humidifier you choose, you should clean it regularly, and it's a good idea to control it with a *humidistat* so it will turn on and off automatically. In the winter, if you notice moisture condensing on windows, or if mold is starting to grow on walls (cold corners and closets are particularly vulnerable) there's too much moisture in the air. To avoid the various problems associated with humidifiers, you might simply drink more water, use a skin moisturizer, or mist the air with distilled water instead.

52. Can dehumidifiers also be unhealthy?

Air conditioners and dehumidifiers both pull moisture from the air, making it more comfortable and less likely to result in mold growth or, in severe cases, rot. Too much humidity can also cause formaldehyde and other VOCs (#6) to outgas faster.

In general, dehumidifiers are less of a problem than humidifiers, but they usually have a container that fills with water that must be emptied and cleaned regularly. When the contain is full of water, it can be susceptible to bacterial growth. A good solution is to get a unit that can be hooked up to a floor drain with a piece of tubing. That way, there's nothing to empty. Actually, most of the time, dehumidifiers solve more problems than they cause.

Dehumidifiers are often used to deal with a mold problem in a basement. When properly constructed, conditioned, and ventilated, a basement should be dry. However, many basements aren't properly constructed, conditioned, or ventilated—so they're damp and moldy. If this is the case in your basement, you should first carefully analyze just why it's so damp, then try to fix any problems. For example, your gutters might be dumping too much rain water next to the house, there may be broken or clogged drainage tiles, or an older basement may have no dampproof coating. The basement may also be too cool (high relative humidity can be more of a problem when the air is cool) or poorly ventilated. If you decide that repairs are too costly, a dehumidifier may be the most cost-effective option. There don't appear to be any health-related differences between various models, but some have more capacity that others, and some are noisier.

53. Which is healthier for bathtubs and showers–acrylic or fiberglass?

Actually, steel and cast-iron tubs are the most inert because they have a porcelainized finish. But, when a tub is also to have a shower, you need to have some type of waterproof wall covering. Ceramic tile can be inert, but the grout lines often get moldy. So, many mold-sensitive people opt for a one-piece tub/shower combination because there are no seams for mold to grow. Both acrylic and fiberglass models are fabricated of synthetic materials, but the fiberglass models seem to be slightly less bothersome.

We usually recommend that they be purchased early and be allowed to air out before installing them.

The frames around shower doors are notorious for getting moldy. A good solution is to use what are called *frameless* shower doors. They have an aluminum frame that mounts to the shower walls, but the glass doors themselves have no framing. Instead, the glass has easy-to-keep-clean polished edges. Most also have a free-draining lower track that's also easy to clean.

54. Is there a healthy bathtub caulking?

For general purpose caulking in bathrooms (and also in kitchens), we like Dap Kwik-Seal Tub and Tile Caulk. It's widely available in hardware stores, building-supply centers, and lumberyards. It contains a mild fungicide—which is important in damp areas—but seems to outgas fairly quickly. In fact, we've found that most sensitive people tolerate it within 4-5 days of application.

VII.
Electrical wiring

VII.

55. What are electromagnetic fields?

Electromagnetic fields, or EMFs for short, are invisible areas of energy. There are actually many different kinds. EMFs can be found around gamma rays, X-rays, ultraviolet light, visible light, infrared radiation, and radio waves. However, the kind most people are concerned about are the EMFs surrounding electrical wiring and appliances.

Anything that uses electricity will be surrounded with electromagnetic fields, of which there are two types—magnetic fields and electric fields. Just plugging something in will cause it have an electric field around it, but it must be operating (current must be flowing) to have a magnetic field.

Most researchers believe that electric fields are relatively benign, and that health effects are more likely to be related to magnetic fields. Magnetic fields are measured in units called milliGauss (mG), but there aren't any well-established guidelines as to how much is too much. Still, it's believed by most researchers that you should stay away from long-term exposures above 3 mG.

56. Can electrical appliances and the wiring inside my walls make me sick?

In most cases, probably not—but there are certainly situations where you should be concerned. The most common health effect researchers are looking into is cancer, but the evidence is often conflicting. In electrical occupations (electricians, linemen, etc.), some forms of cancer are seen more often than in workers who aren't routinely around high-strength fields. And, some studies have found leukemia more often in people who live near high-voltage power lines.

There are three factors that determine how harmful an EMF exposure is: the strength of the field, your distance from the field, and your exposure time. Being near a high-strength field for many hours at a time is believed to be more serious than being near a high-strength field for a few minutes, or a low-strength field for an extended period of time.

To know for sure how strong a field is, you must measure it with a special device called a Gaussmeter. Gaussmeters are available from several mail-order companies, such as N.E.E.D.S. (527 Charles Ave. #12-A, Syracuse, NY 13209, 800-634-1380) and Nontoxic Environments, Inc. (P.O. Box 384, New Market, NH 03857, 800-789-4348). Fields vary considerably from one appliance to another, and they fluctuate at different times of the day. For example on a hot summer day, when everyone is using their air conditioner, there will stronger fields under outdoor power lines than on a cool fall evening when less electricity is being used.

You can often measure magnetic fields in the hundreds of mG very close to small electrical appliances (shavers, hair dryers, hand mixers, etc.). However, you don't use these devices for hours on end, and the fields are often fairly weak a foot or so away. This is an important point to keep in mind—all electromagnetic fields get weaker as you move away from their source.

There can be high-strength magnetic fields around fluorescent-light ballasts, dimmer switches, power panels, electric heaters, electric stoves, TVs, computer monitors, and motors. Areas of high-strength fields are often called *electromagnetic hot spots*. One way to avoid very much exposure is to position furniture (especially beds) at a distance where the fields are reduced. In most homes, the hot spots only have a high-strength field that extends outward for a foot or two.

Magnetic fields are difficult to block. In fact, they're rarely affected by walls. So, if you measure an electromagnetic hot spot near your refrigerator, you should consider what's directly behind it on the opposite side of the partition wall. This is an important consideration that's sometimes overlooked.

If you live near high-voltage power lines, or an electrical substation, you can often have your electric utility measure the fields for you. They generally won't measure the fields *inside* your home, and they usually contend that EMFs aren't a health problem. But, they often get a lot of phone calls about EMFs, so they usually have meters to measure fields around their own equipment. Where power lines are a problem, some people have moved their bed into a different bedroom—further away from the power lines to minimize their risk.

If you have electric radiant heat in your ceiling or if you have outdated knob-and-tube wiring in your house, they can bathe entire rooms in high-strength EMFs. Electric blankets can also be a problem, but most manufacturers have redesigned their products to have lower-strength fields than in the past. For more information about EMFs (and other indoor-air-quality issues), you can call the Environmental Health Clearing-house at 800-643-4794.

57. Is it true that metal plumbing lines can contribute an EMF problem?

Yes, in some houses, this can be true. Electrical codes require that metal plumbing lines be grounded to minimize the danger of electrical shock. This is important, and an excellent thing to do. However, there are situations where the plumb-ing lines (or natural-gas lines) can actually be carrying a small amount of electricity. If this is the case, the metal pipes can be surrounded by mag-netic fields.

These situations can be difficult to diagnose and fix, but it can be done (#58). One thing that's important to remember—you should never remove any plumbing-line grounding connections.

58. Can my house have an EMF problem because of something in my neighbor's house?

That can occur. It usually happens when there's a water-pipe grounding problem in one house (#57), and two or more houses are interconnected by underground metal pipes. In some cases, high-strength EMFs throughout a neighborhood can be traced to a single problem in one house.

Electricians wishing to learn how to diagnose and solve EMF-grounding problems should get a copy of the book *Tracing EMFs in Building Wiring and Grounding* by Karl Riley.

59. What are some simple ways to minimize EMFs?

When you're planning to build a new house, you should test the background EMF level on your site—if there are any power lines, substations, or transformers nearby. If high levels are found, you may want to reposition the house elsewhere on the lot. When the house is being wired, don't locate the meter, power panels, or major power cables near the bedrooms because that's where you'll be spending eight hours or so at a time. Make sure your home is properly grounded, and there is no current flowing on the water pipes. Because many appliances have high-strength fields, the easiest thing to do with them is to step away while they are operating. For example, you may want to sit further away from your computer monitor, or move your clock radio to the other side of your night stand so it isn't right next to your head.

Remember, all houses have electromagnetic hot spots. The goal is not to eliminate all of them. Rather, it's to locate them in parts of the home where you don't spend a great deal of time. For example, even though you might walk by a power panel in a hallway several times a day, that's better than having it next to your head while you're sleeping in bed.

60. What is electromagnetic sensitivity?

Recently, the term *electromagnetic sensitivity* has emerged. People with this condition are negatively affected by EMFs at lower field strengths than the rest of us. They sometimes report dizziness, ringing in the ears, muscle weakness, confusion, fainting, or other symptoms. Electromagnetic sensitivity doesn't seem to be as common as chemical sensitivity, but some people are affected by both. *The Electromagnetic Sensitivity Handbook* by Lucinda Grant is a good source for information on this condition.

61. What can an electromagnetically sensitive person do to make his or her home safer?

Unfortunately, some people with electromagnetic sensitivity have had to avoid electricity completely. However, many get relief by reducing their exposure considerably. For example, they may sit further away from their computer screen than they did previously. Some have reverted to using a manual typewriter. One thing that often helps is to turn off the circuit breaker at the power panel that serves the bedroom before going to bed. If you do this, make sure you aren't accidentally turning something important off—like the refrigerator.

62. Can't metal siding on a house cause EMF problems?

This is something we're asked about quite often even though, as it turns out, it's unlikely to be a problem. The idea dates back to 1980, when a book dealing with indoor pollution said that a metal-sided house would act like a Faraday cage and interfere with a person's natural biologic rhythms—such as their waking/sleep pattern.

A Faraday cage is a special room that electrical technicians sometimes use to evaluate equipment or perform tests in. It usually has well-grounded metal screen on all sides, top, and bottom, and it's designed to block out all forms of radiation. As a result, there's no electrical interference of any kind inside the room.

If a person spends an extended period of time in a Faraday cage (several days or a few weeks), their body gets out-of-sync and their natural rhythms start functioning differently. This is because a Faraday cage blocks out the weak naturally occurring background electromagnetic radiation that regulates our systems. The human species has been surrounded by this natural beneficial radiation for tens-of-thousands of years.

While a metal-sided house may, at first, seem like a Faraday cage, it really isn't. In fact, it would be very difficult for a home to duplicate the same conditions inside a real Faraday cage. For example, there couldn't be any windows, doors, or other openings. In addition, all the individual pieces of metal siding would need to be soldered together, there would need to be a metal roof and a metal floor, and everything would need to be securely grounded. Even if all that was done, a person would need to remain indoors, because going outside would cause their rhythms to be restored.

63. I'm bothered by the odor of plastics. Will plastic-jacketed electrical wiring be a problem for me?

It could be—especially if you're directly exposed to new wire. It's possible to minimize outgassing by running the wiring inside metal conduit—but this isn't often done in residences because it can be expensive. What we recommend is to buy the wiring early in the construction process and let it air out before it's installed. Some people have had it sitting in a garage for several months while other work is being done on the house.

Once the walls are covered with wallboard, the wiring isn't exposed to the living space. So, it usually isn't a problem. But for sensitive people—just to be extra safe—we usually suggest that it be wrapped with household aluminum foil to reduce outgassing inside the walls.

VIII.
Heating and cooling

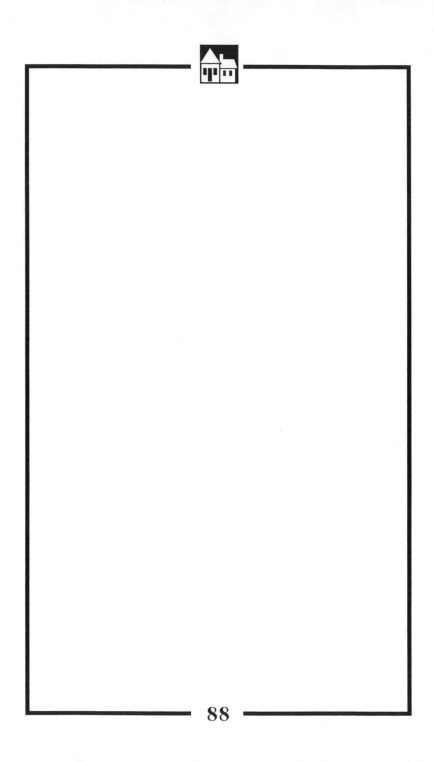

VIII.

64. Why don't you like fireplaces or gas ranges?

Actually, we don't like most fuel-burning appliances—fireplaces, wood stoves, gas ranges, oil furnaces, space heaters, water heaters, boilers, etc. Many people think the reason we don't like them has to do fuel leaks. While oil or gas leaks certainly can pollute a house, we're much more concerned with poor chimney function. Whenever you burn something, you have combustion by-products with which to contend. And, it isn't healthy to have any combustion by-products indoors. The worst offenders are unvented appliances because they have no chimney whatsoever, and they dump combustion by-products directly into the indoor air.

You might think that if a fuel-burning device is connected to a chimney, the situation would be better. Well, in many cases it is—but in many cases it isn't. You see, chimneys don't always function correctly. The combustion by-products (which are warm) rise up through a chimney because warm air rises. You can actually measure a slight upward pressure (called a draft) inside a chimney. Problems occur when there's a negative pressure (that wants to pull in) within the living space that's greater than the draft pressure (that wants to push up and out). If that's the case, air can come down the chimney, and the combustion by-products can't go up. When this occurs, they spill into the living space.

If there's a complete reversal of flow in a chimney (downward), it's called *backdrafting*, and all the combustion by-products enter the house. In many cases, the draft is only partially affected, and some combustion by-products go up the chimney while some enter the living space. This situation is called *spillage*.

Backdrafting and spillage are actually quite common. In some houses they're regular occurrences. For example, we've all smelled wood smoke indoors—smoke that should've gone up the chimney. Experts estimate that 50-80% of chimneys have the potential to malfunction.

Sometimes chimneys don't work because of poor design, lack of maintenance, or damage. But, an increasing problem has to do with very small air pressure differences. A typical draft pressure in a chimney is often less than 5 Pascals (Pa.). A Pa. is a tiny unit of air pressure. (There are over 200,000 Pa. of pressure in an automobile tire.) If any device is blowing air outdoors, it can cause a very slight negative pressure in the entire house. (Exhaust fans, clothes dryers, and central vacuums have all been implicated.) If that slight negative pressure is more than 5 Pa., you can have chimney problems. There are a number of factors that come into play (house tightness, temperature, wind conditions, etc.), but a Canadian study found that about half of all houses would have a problem if a typical

kitchen-range exhaust and clothes dryer were
operating at the same time..

65. What's so bad about combustion by-products?

Different fuels release different combustion
by-products, but none are good to have indoors.
Wood smoke may have a pleasant aroma, but it
probably isn't any better for you to breathe than
tobacco smoke. Common combustion by-products
include carbon dioxide, carbon monoxide, formaldehyde, nitrogen oxides, particulates, sulfur oxide,
water vapor, and various hydrocarbons. Some are
worse than others.

For example, carbon dioxide isn't particularly
dangerous—at least not in the concentrations typically found in houses. While water vapor doesn't
sound too bad, it can certainly cause problems.
That's because burning a pound of fuel can release
almost a pound of water vapor. If backdrafting or
spillage are chronic problems, enough water vapor
can enter the living space to cause mold or mildew
growth.

Carbon monoxide is colorless and odorless
and is, by far, one of the worst pollutants found
indoors. The reason for this is, it's particularly deadly
at fairly low concentrations. Several hundred Americans die each year indoors due to carbon-monoxide
poisoning. Fortunately, most cases aren't serious
enough to kill people. But, low-level carbon-monoxide
poisoning seems to be a very common cause of flu-
like symptoms such as nausea, malaise, headache,

etc. In one study, 24% of people who thought they had the flu didn't. They were actually being poisoned by exposure to a low level of carbon monoxide.

It's been found that over 19% of the children in wood-heated homes have allergies, compared to only about 3% in houses with other forms of heat. Wheezing and coughing are also more common in wood-heated homes. Think your gas range is OK? Think again. There are studies showing that children are more likely to have respiratory symptoms if gas is used for cooking, and women who cook with gas have a significant increase in symptoms such as wheezing, waking with shortness of breath, and asthma attacks. They're also twice as likely to have impaired lung function than women who cook with electric stoves.

66. Are there any fuel-burning appliances that are safer than others?

Actually, there are some that are quite good. These all have one thing in common—they have *totally sealed combustion chambers.* Here's what happens inside a regular gas furnace (or boiler, or water heater): air moves from the living space into an open combustion chamber, where the gas and air mix, and are burned. Then, the combustion by-products rise out of the chamber up into a chimney and leave the house.

Here's how a sealed-combustion gas furnace works: air is pulled from the outdoors through a sealed intake pipe, into a sealed combustion chamber, where it mixes with the gas and burns. Then, the combustion by-products are blown outdoors by a fan through a sealed exhaust pipe. The entire process is sealed, an exhaust pipe is used instead of a chimney, and there's no way combustion by-products can enter the living space (unless something is broken).

Most major furnace producers offer high-efficiency sealed-combustion gas furnaces. There are also sealed-combustion water heaters and sealed-combustion boilers—if you have hot-water heating. Plus, most gas-fireplace manufacturers offer at least one sealed-combustion model. Sealed-combustion gas fireplaces are often called *direct-vent* fireplaces. If you plan to use gas for heating, we believe sealed-combustion appliances are the only way to go.

67. Are electric furnaces and water heaters inherently healthier?

Electric furnaces operate somewhat like a toaster. They contain a heating element that warms the air. Electric boilers and water heaters also contain heating elements. Electricity is convenient to use—but it can be an expensive way to heat a house, or to heat water.

Heat pumps use electricity more efficiently, so they're often more cost-effective. Plus, they can provide both heat in the winter and air conditioning in the summer. Some heat pumps have an outdoor unit that pulls heat from the air. Geothermal heat pumps pull heat from the earth. Heat-pump water heaters are also available.

Electric appliances are sort of a mixed bless-ing. Their biggest health advantage is there are no combustion by-products. But it should be remem-bered, combustion by-products aren't a problem with sealed-combustion appliances either (#66). Although in most cases fuel leaks aren't as serious a problem as combustion by-products, electric appliances will never leak any fuel. But, they can be surrounded by electromagnetic fields (#55).

68. What's the best type of heat for a sensitive person?

Sensitive people can react to all kinds of things that aren't bothersome to healthy people. For example, if dust falls on a hot surface in a furnace or on a radiator it can burn. Granted, this isn't a serious issue for most people, but the tiny amounts of combustion by-products released by burning dust can bother some who are sensitive. Certain individuals have even been known to react to the small amount of odor released by a warm fan motor in a furnace.

We've found that hot-water heating is a good choice for sensitive people. Sometimes just one boiler can serve radiators, a radiant-heating system in the floor, and also provide hot water for all your indoor needs.

Nordyne (1801 Park 270 Dr. #600, St. Louis, MO 63146, 800-422-4328) makes self-contained Intertherm-brand baseboard heaters that are often well tolerated. We've used them successfully in several houses for sensitive people. They have a

metal case with an inert baked-enamel finish. However, some people have had to run them for 2-3 days
on high heat to burn off any minor contaminants.
They run on electricity, so they can be expensive to
operate if you live in a cold climate and your house
isn't particularly well insulated.

69. Is using duct tape a good idea?

Sealing duct joints is a very good idea, but
duct tape isn't the best material to use. In the not-too-
distant past, sheet-metal ductwork was assembled
with a few sheet-metal screws, and nothing special
was done to the joints between the different pieces.
Then, people started sealing the joints with duct
tape—only to find that it didn't last very long. In some
cases, duct tape (even the more-expensive aluminum-foil type) falls off after less than a year.

Most experts now recommend using *duct-
sealing mastics*. They're much more durable and
longer lasting than tape. We prefer the water-based
versions. They're about the consistency of mashed
potatoes. We've applied them in a number of ways
including smearing on a joint with a gloved hand,
using a brush, and troweling.

Sealing ducts is a good idea for several
reasons. For example, sealed ducts are more energy
efficient. It isn't unusual to find that 20% of the air is
leaking into, or out of, a typical duct system. If the
ducts are in an attic or crawl space, then you're
blowing air into and sucking it out of those spaces—
rather than moving all of it into and out of the living
space. Leaky ducts can also be unhealthy. There are

many cases where particles of insulation from an attic, or mold spores from a crawl space, are sucked into leaky ducts and blown into the living space. Leaky ducts can also cause enough of a pressure imbalance in a house to result in backdrafting or spillage (#64).

70. Should heating/cooling ducts be cleaned occasionally?

You're going to be breathing the air that passes through your ducts. So if they're dirty, they should probably be cleaned. Some ducts get very dirty very quickly, but others remain relatively clean for years. If ducts are leaky, they can suck pollutants into them. If the living space is polluted, airborne contaminants can be pulled into ducts with the air that's to be heated or cooled. All this dirty air can coat the inside of the ducts—if there isn't a good filter to capture it.

Most major cities have duct-cleaning services listed in the telephone directory. They typically use a high-powered truck-mounted vacuum connected to a long hose that's snaked through the ducts to suck out any dirt and debris. Some systems use rotating brushes, and some operators like to spray the inside of the cleaned ducts with a disinfectant or sealer. In general, we feel cleaning ducts periodically can be a good idea. However, we don't like the idea of spraying any kind of chemical into them. Just stick with the vacuuming.

In the last few years, a product called *ductboard* has become very widely used instead of sheet-metal ducts. We don't like it at all because its fiberglass lining is directly exposed to the airstream. As a result, it can contaminate the air you'll be breathing with glass fibers, as well as with outgassing from the formaldehyde-based resin. Ductboard is also virtually impossible to clean. Round, flexible, plastic-lined ducts are also popular today. They don't outgas very much, but sensitive people often special-order them with an aluminum-foil inner liner.

71. What are the advantages and disadvantages to ductless heating and cooling systems?

Hot-water heating systems don't have the problems associated with leaky or dirty ducts. Plus they can be quieter, and many people prefer the fact that air isn't being blown around. Radiantly heated concrete or ceramic-tile floors are very popular because they feel warm to walk on. Although they aren't common, some radiators can be used for cooling by running chilled water through them.

Several companies make small wall-mounted air-conditioners (or heat pumps) that use no duct work. These *mini-split systems* have an indoor unit that hangs on a wall, and an outdoor unit that looks similar to that used with a conventional central air conditioner. They can be very effective in an existing house where ductwork would be difficult to install.

The big disadvantage to ductless heating and cooling systems is the fact that they can't be fitted with air filters. While most forced-air heating/cooling systems really don't have very good filters, at least you have the option of adding one. In reality, you can't always avoid ducts completely because, if you're interested in ventilation—and we think you should be—it will usually require some.

IX.
Ventilation

IX.

72. Exactly what is ventilation anyway?

Simply put, ventilation is the *exchange* of air in a house. In other words, it means bringing in fresh air and expelling stale, polluted, moisture-laden air.

73. My attic is vented, so my house is adequately ventilated, right?

Actually, no. Attic ventilation is for attics, and crawl space ventilation is for crawl spaces. What we're talking about is ventilation for the living space, because that's where people are.

We're often asked about ceiling fans. They're designed to *circulate* air within a room—not to exchange the indoor and outdoor air. So, they aren't considered ventilation fans. They may help make you feel comfortable, but they don't remove pollutants or moisture from the house.

74. Why is ventilating houses so important?

Nearly all homes contain building materials, furnishings, decorating items, and cleaning products that outgas pollutants into the indoor air. Ventilation can dilute the concentration of those pollutants. But, even if totally inert, safe alternatives are used, there's one pollution source that can't be eliminated—people. Because of normal, everyday human metabolism, we all release various gases such as carbon dioxide, water vapor, ammonia, methane, etc. If allowed to build up indoors, these can make a house odorous and uncomfortable. Plus, we all need a supply of fresh air indoors to replace the oxygen that gets used up.

If you have an unhealthy house (one built, maintained, and furnished with unhealthy materials), you'll probably need a powerful (and expensive) ventilation system to dilute the concentration of all the indoor pollutants. But if you have a healthy house, the ventilation system's primary job will be to dilute the metabolic pollutants released by the occupants—so it doesn't need to be as powerful. In other words, most houses need ventilation systems, but healthy houses often get by with less powerful, inexpensive ones.

75. Can't a house breathe naturally– like people do?

This is a real common question. In fact, we do think houses should breathe—but they can't possible do it the same way as human beings. People breathe through specific orifices (nose and mouth) because certain muscles (the diaphragm) cause lungs to expand and contract. Houses have no muscles and they can't expand and contract, so they must breathe differently. Airplanes fly differently than birds, and houses breathe differently than people.

We're strong believers in mechanical ventilation. That means using one or more fans (usually small ones) to exchange the indoor air for outdoor air.

76. Why not just build a loose house?

In loose houses, there's a certain amount of air exchange caused by Mother Nature. For example, when the wind blows on the side of a house, it pushes air through the cracks into the living space. At the same time, air will be leaving through cracks in the opposite side of the house.

Sometimes a loose house works just fine, but there are several disadvantages. First of all, with a loosely built house, you have no control over how much air is entering and leaving—or where it's entering and leaving. If the wind isn't blowing, there may be almost no air exchange. At other times, there may be far more than you need. With this feast-or-famine approach, you typically get far too much ventilation in the middle of winter when the incoming air is very cold, uncomfortable, and expensive to heat.

When air is leaking in through the cracks of a loose house, it will be unfiltered. Therefore, whatever pollutants exist outdoors (smoke, overspray from lawn chemicals, pollen, etc.) will be brought inside. In addition, particles and gases from insulation can be pulled into the living space, and moisture can leak into building cavities—contributing to a hidden mold problem or rot.

There have been a number of studies that have measured how much air enters houses naturally due to certain factors, such as the wind. What they've found is that houses are much tighter than they used to be, and as a result, they often don't get enough natural ventilation to satisfy the basic needs of the occupants.

The solution is not to build looser houses, because loose houses are drafty, uncomfortable, too dry in the winter, and expensive to heat and cool. There are good reasons to build tight houses (#37), and if they're ventilated mechanically, you can have comfort, energy efficiency, and health—the best of all worlds.

77. Are there different kinds of ventilation?

Yes, there are two basic kinds—*local* ventilation and *general* ventilation—and most houses will benefit from both. Local ventilation is designed to remove large amounts of pollution or moisture quickly. Many homes already have local ventilation in the forms of kitchen-range exhausts and bathroom exhaust fans. These fans are typically used only occasionally. Bath fans are turned on to remove moisture after a steamy shower, or to eliminate toilet odors. Kitchen fans expel moisture and cooking odors. By using local ventilation as necessary, excess moisture and pollution are prevented from spreading throughout the house.

General ventilation is designed to exchange the air in the entire house slowly. It's important because people don't confine themselves to one room—they move throughout the house. And wherever they go, they need oxygen. They also need fresh air to dilute their metabolic by-products (#74). If your house is reasonably healthy, there are some basic guidelines that have been established to determine how much general ventilation you need. In most cases, 15 cubic feet of air per minute (cfm) is enough for each person. Another rule-of thumb suggests you calculate the volume of the house (all the indoor space) and use a ventilation rate that will exchange $\frac{1}{3}$ of the air every hour.

78. What kinds of ventilation equipment are available?

Ventilation equipment falls into three basic categories: *depressurization* systems, *pressurization* systems, and *balanced* systems. Bath fans and kitchen-range hoods are almost always exhaust fans. When they blow stale, polluted air outdoors, the house becomes slightly depressurized, and an equal volume of *make-up air* enters somewhere else. If you have a loosely built house, the make-up air will enter through the cracks. But in a tight house, you may need to poke one or more holes in a wall for the make-up air to enter. At first, this may seem ridiculous—build a tight house, then deliberately poke some holes in it. However, it's really much better than having a loose house because, if you install the holes, you have control over how much air is entering, where it's entering, and where it's leaving. Plus, it's usually more energy efficient.

You can also use an exhaust fan for general ventilation. For example, you might have a single fan hooked to some ductwork to pull stale air from several rooms at once. This approach is usually combined with deliberate holes in the walls of several rooms so the make-up air can enter. Several companies sell *make-up air inlets* (often called *through-the-wall vents*) which are designed to allow a specific amount of air to enter. They're often placed in bedrooms, or other rooms, where it's nice to have a continuous supply of incoming fresh air. If you opt for this approach, you should know that make-up air inlets are equipped with very inefficient filters.

All exhaust fans slightly *depressurize* a house, something that can interfere with chimney function (#64). (Of course, if your house doesn't have a chimney, this may not be a concern.) It's also possible to use a fan to blow fresh air indoors—which will slightly *pressurizes* a house. In a tight house that's pressurized, through-the-wall vents are necessary to allow stale air to escape. While pressurization systems are possible, they aren't common. In cold climates, pressurization usually isn't a good idea because it can push excess moisture from the living space into wall cavities. This can result in hidden condensation, mold growth, or rot.

Balanced ventilation systems use two fans—one to blow fresh air indoors and one to blow stale air outdoors. As long as the airflows are equal, this approach neither pressurizes nor depressurizes the house. The incoming and outgoing air is often ducted to different rooms. Because this approach requires two fans, the equipment can be more expensive to purchase and operate. However, it can give you the most control and provide better distribution of the air. In cold climates, there's a specialized type of balanced ventilator that's become popular. It's called a *heat recovery ventilator*. It's actually the most common type of general ventilation equipment on the market.

79. What exactly is a heat recovery ventilator?

Although the terms have slightly different meanings, most *heat recovery ventilators* (HRVs), are also called *air-to-air heat exchangers*. They're balanced ventilators. So basically, they consist of a sheet-metal cabinet with two fans. But, they also have a special heat-recovery core. During operation, the incoming fresh air and the outgoing stale air pass very close to each other inside the core. They don't touch and contaminate each other. However, the heat from the warmer airstream passes through the core into the colder airstream, warming it up. So, in the winter with an HRV, the outgoing stale air warms up the incoming fresh air. This makes HRVs more energy efficient than other forms of ventilation.

There are different kinds of HRVs available. Some have different types of cores (rotary, heat-pipe, or flat plate) which are made of different materials (metal, paper, or plastic). Their efficiency varies depending on the specific design features. When shopping for one, ask about ease of cleaning, whether it has an automatic defrosting system, its capacity, control options, what special features it has, what materials were used in its construction, and cost.

80. Isn't ventilation equipment expensive?

Well, it certainly costs something. If you want a healthy house, we feel ventilation is a necessary expense. Fortunately, the cost doesn't have to be exorbitant. In fact, there's a wide variety of equipment available. Some is inexpensive to install but more costly to operate. The actual operating expenses will depend on the cost of electricity, the harshness of the climate, how powerful the ventilator is, and how often you run it.

If you opt for an HRV you'll spend more up-front on equipment, but your operating cost will be lower. The cheapest general ventilation system might only cost a couple of hundred dollars to install. On the other hand, a Cadillac system with all the bells and whistles could run as much as $3,000 by the time it's all hooked up. There's really something for every budget.

In most parts of the U.S., the operating cost of a general ventilation system is routinely in the neighborhood of $100 per year, and it's often less. While HRVs can be costly to purchase, they can pay for themselves in energy savings in a few years—if you're in a very cold climate. If you live in a mild climate, HRVs generally aren't cost effective, so other strategies can make more sense. When all the costs are factored in, it's usually cheaper to build a tight house with a mechanical ventilation system than a loose house that's ventilated (often overventilated) haphazardly by Mother Nature.

X.
Air filters

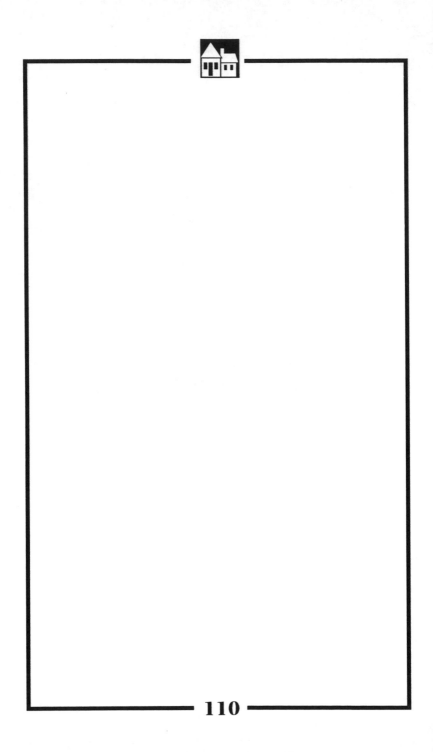

X.

81. Won't a good air filter remove all the pollution in my house?

In most cases, filtration isn't the single answer, but it can be part of the answer. To have good indoor air quality, you first need to apply the three Healthy-House Design Principles of eliminate, separate, and ventilate (#12). Once that's been done, the indoor air should be pretty good, and you can use a filter to remove any minor pollutants that are left. A good filter is not a substitute for ventilation because filters can't remove moisture from the air and they can't supply oxygen.

If you want to try and use filtration to clean up the air in a problem house, you'll need a very powerful system that will filter the air several times an hour. This will be expensive, breezy, and noisy, and it won't be as effective as applying the three Healthy-House Design Principles first.

If you decide to use a filter, there are three ways to do so. First, you can use a portable room-sized filter. There are a number of companies that offer these free-standing units. Mail-order suppliers include Allermed Corp. (31 Steel Rd., Wylie, TX 75098, 214-442-4898), E.L. Foust Co. (P.O. Box 105, Elmhurst, IL 60126, 800-225-9549), and N.E.E.D.S. (527 Charles Ave. #12-A, Syracuse, NY 13209, 800-634-1380).

Portable filters work best in a single room, with the door closed, and the filter left running continuously. Second, for whole-house filtration, you can let the fan on your forced-air furnace or central air conditioner run continuously so its filter will remove pollutants passing through the system. Third, you can use a filter with a general ventilation system to filter the incoming air—air that isn't always as clean as we'd like it to be. In some cases, it can make sense to combine a forced-air heating/cooling system with a ventilation system. That way, one filter (and one set of ducts) can serve both systems.

82. My furnace already has a filter. Isn't that good enough?

This is a common misconception. Furnace filters are *furnace* filters—not *people* filters. They exist primarily to remove very large particles that can damage the bearings in a fan motor, or clog the coil in a central air conditioner. People need much more efficient filtration.

83. I've seen ads offering filters that are 90% efficient. Are they any good?

While there are hundreds of different pollutants, from a filtration standpoint, they can be placed in two categories—particulates (small particles) and gases. You need a particulate filter to remove particulates and a gas filter to remove gases. There isn't a standardized way to evaluate gas filters, but there's more than one way to measure particulate-filter efficiency—and this leads to some misleading advertising and a great deal of confusion.

Particulate-filter efficiency is most-often measured with either an *Arrestance* test or an *Atmospheric Spot-Dust* test. Both are described in detail in a technical standard called ASHRAE 52-76. The Arrestance test really isn't very useful because it only measures how well a filter captures large particulates—something all filters do fairly well. For example, a standard 1"-thick furnace filter is about 80% efficient when measured on an Arrestance test. For most residential applications, it's better to use the Spot-Dust test—on which a standard furnace filter is only 3-5% efficient.

So, to answer the question, a filter that's 90% efficient on an Arrestance test isn't nearly as good as a filter that's 90% efficient on a Spot-Dust test. We routinely see ads for 90%-efficient filters, and many use the Arrestance test (although they rarely say so on the ad). They're certainly better than a standard furnace filter, but not as efficient as you might think.

84. What are the different types of air filters, and how efficient are they?

Electrostatic air filters are made of plastic that's manufactured to hold a charge of static electricity. Because of this charge, particulate pollutants cling to the filter. It's the same principle that causes some clothing to cling. These filters are often advertised as being 90% efficient. When they're evaluated on a Spot-Dust test (#83), they're 10-15% efficient. While that may not sound like much, it's 3-4 times as good as a standard furnace filter. These filters actually do a reasonable job with most larger mold and pollen particles. They're not too expensive, and they can be easily installed in an existing forced-air heating/cooling system. Some can be cleaned and reused, but others must be replaced when they get dirty. Filtrete is one popular brand made by 3M, but there are several others.

Electrostatic precipitators also operate with static electricity, but they require an electric current to function. They're commonly called *electronic air cleaners*, and are widely available through heating/cooling contractors. They have electrical wires inside them that cause particulates to become charged, and collector plates that capture the charged particulates. When these filters are clean, they're typically an impressive 90% efficient on a Spot-Dust test. But, as the collector plates fill with dust, they lose more and more efficiency. It isn't unusual for the efficiency to drop to 20% in just a few days if the air in a house is very dusty. They're easy to clean—you just slide the filter unit out of its housing, and place it in a dishwasher. Manufacturers usually recommend washing them at least once a month—but some people find that cleaning is necessary every week. There's nothing to replace with these filters, but they do produce a small amount of ozone during normal operation (#85).

Extended-surface air filters are 2-6" thick, and they're made in a pleated, accordion-like shape. This gives them a great deal of surface area—something that's important to minimize the resistance to airflow. Space-Gard is a popular brand with which heating/cooling contractors are usually familiar, but there are several others that are similar. Because of their thickness, they must be installed in a special housing in the furnace/air-conditioning ductwork. They typically last for a year or two depending on how dirty the air is, and preform at 25-45% efficiency on a Spot-Dust test. This is good enough to capture most common mold spores and pollen particles, so these filters work very well for many allergy sufferers. However, the filter itself is made of fiberglass or polyester fibers held together with a resin, and some sensitive people are bothered by the minor odor of the resin.

HEPA (high efficiency particulate accumulator) filters are extremely efficient. They typically register 98% or higher on a Spot-Dust test, but they're usually evaluated with an even-more-accurate DOP-Smoke-Penetration test. A HEPA filter is actually a specialized kind of extended-surface filter. In order to minimize the resistance to airflow through them (which can be considerable), they're usually several inches thick. For residential heating/cooling systems, you must use a more-powerful fan motor just to get very much air to move through these filters. HEPAs are the most efficient particulate filters you can buy. They were originally developed for use in atomic-energy labs to filter out tiny plutonium particles. While it's a good idea to remove as many particulates as possible from the air, in most residential applications, HEPAs are really often overkill. They can also have a slight odor that bothers some sensitive people.

All the filters mentioned so far are designed to capture particulates. To remove gases from the air, you must use an adsorption (spelled with a D) material, of which activated carbon is the most widely used. When a gas such as formaldehyde passes through an adsorption filter, it clings (adheres) to it. After a while, the adsorption material can't hold any more gas molecules, and the filter must be replaced. Activated alumina (brand names include Purafil and Carusorb) is another adsorption material, and it actually does a better job of capturing formaldehyde than activated carbon. For these filters to be effective, and to last more than a few days, they generally need a considerable amount of adsorption material. The best filters weigh at least several pounds, but there are some on the market that only contain a few ounces of activated-carbon dust. The heavier filters can have a great deal of resistance to airflow, and they can't be easily adapted to residential applications—unless the fan motor is replaced with a more-powerful model.

If you're very sensitive and want a very efficient filtration system, you should know that all filters add something to the air that wasn't there before. They typically remove far more than they add, but sensitive people can react negatively to the filter itself. For example, the slight odor of an electrostatic air filter, an extended-surface filter, or a HEPA filter really isn't an issue for most people. However, it can bother some sensitive persons. So can the ozone from an electrostatic precipitator, and some people are bothered by activated carbon manufactured from coal but not carbon made from coconut shells.

While it's fairly easy to get most of the whole-house filters we've discussed through heating/cooling contractors, it's more difficult to locate a residential supplier of adsorption filters containing very much material, or HEPA filters. If you're interested in these approaches, Allermed Corp. (31 Steel Rd., Wylie, TX 75098, 214-442-4898) and Pure Air Systems, Inc. (P.O. Box 418, Plainfield, IN 46168, 800-869-8025) make units that can be used with a residential forced-air heating/cooling system.

85. Several people have told me to get an ozone generator. What do you think?

In most cases, we don't think they're a good idea. Ozone is a very-well-studied air pollutant that can cause eye, nose, and lung inflammation. When there's a smog alert in a major city and people are told to stay indoors, it's because ozone levels are high. So why, you might ask, are ozone generators being sold as a solution to indoor air pollution problems? Well, it's because manufacturers have taken a grain of truth and stretched it.

There's evidence ozone can chemically react with some VOCs and the end product of the reaction is water vapor and carbon dioxide—two innocuous compounds. However, this reaction takes place slowly. In the meantime, the ozone can be reacting negatively with your lungs. Ozone can also kill bacteria and mold. But, if it's strong enough to that, it's not doing you any good either. In some cases, ozone can react with pollutants in the air and form new bothersome compounds that weren't there before.

Minnesota, North Carolina, Florida, and California have all come down hard on ozone-generator manufacturers in recent years. These states claim there's no evidence the devices help improve indoor air quality, and they cite a number of reports showing ozone to be harmful to people.

A situation where ozone generators can be helpful is with smoke damage. Ozone has long been known to react with smoky odors and neutralize them. However, ozone should only be used in a smoke-damaged house when it is unoccupied, and the house should be thoroughly aired out before the occupants return.

86. Is a negative-ion generator a filtering device?

Yes and no. A negative-ion generator uses electric current to produce negative ions (free electrons). The ions attach themselves to particulates in the air causing them cling to oppositely charged walls and furnishings. This can result in slightly cleaner air, but dirtier walls. Some negative-ion generators have a built-in filter that captures the charged particulates.

Sometimes these devices are not sold for their filtering ability at all. There are studies showing if there is an overabundance of negative ions in the air, some people can have a feeling of well-being—they just feel better. On the other hand, these devices create a certain amount of ozone (#85) that other people find irritating.

87. Didn't NASA find that house plants could clean the air naturally?

Again, yes and no. In the 1980s, NASA performed a fairly simple experiment. They placed a house plant inside a sealed chamber with a certain amount of formaldehyde. Then, after waiting a while, they measured the concentration of the formaldehyde. Like magic, the formaldehyde was gone. Further research showed that it wasn't the house plants that consumed the formaldehyde—it was specific kinds of bacteria living in the soil in which the plants were growing. Anyway, NASA's simple experiment was widely reported in the press as a revolutionary new idea—house plants as a cure for air pollution. Unfortunately, the real world inside houses is more complicated than the environment inside a NASA test chamber.

In NASA's experiment, a certain quantity of formaldehyde was used. In most houses, there are manufactured wood products which contain a significant reservoir of formaldehyde—enough to release the gas for several years (#10). When plants are in an environment where there's a continuously outgassing source of formaldehyde (either in a house or in a test chamber), several things happen. First, the soil bacteria starts consuming the formaldehyde as food. Then, the formaldehyde source (particle board, or whatever) starts outgassing faster to try to raise the concentration back up to what it was. At the same time, the plant is releasing a certain amount of moisture into the air, and formaldehyde outgases faster as the relative humidity goes up. The net result is a slightly lower concentration of formaldehyde—but not a significant reduction.

This is one of those simple solutions to a complex problem that just doesn't work. Plus, if you have very many plants indoors, the relative humidity can become high enough to result in a mold problem.

XI.
Interior walls

XI.

88. I've heard that plaster is a healthy material. What are its advantages and disadvantages?

You buy plaster as a powder, mix it with water, then apply it to a surface where it hardens. Once completely cured, the plaster is very inert and rock-like. Although most people can't detect any odor after a few days, a few sensitive people have said that they're bothered by a slight odor for a month or so.

In the past, 2-3 coats of plaster were commonly applied on top of thin strips of wood lath. In some commercial applications it's still applied in a similar manner, but it's usually put over to metal lath instead of wood. However, the most common way to use plaster today involves skimming one or two thin coats over a gypsum-board material. The gypsum board has a blue paper face, so it's usually called *blueboard*.

Most of the time, plaster walls are painted. For sensitive people who are bothered by paint, plaster has the advantage of being hard, durable, and scrubbable enough that you can actually leave it unpainted. While most plaster is white, it can sometimes be tinted (before its applied) with the same kinds of mineral pigments that bricklayers use in mortar.

As far as drawbacks, plaster is more brittle than drywall (#89) and, if it ever cracks, it'll no longer be airtight. Plaster costs more than drywall, primarily because of the skilled labor required. In some parts of the country, plaster is widely used. But, in other areas, it's been totally replaced with drywall.

89. What makes drywall different from plaster?

Drywall is a gypsum-board product similar to blueboard (#88). The chief difference has to do with the paper facing. The paper on drywall is a lower-grade paper made from recycled newspaper. Some sensitive people are bothered by printing ink. As a result, they can also be affected by drywall because the paper contains ink residues. This usually isn't a strong pollutant source, and paint often seals the paper well enough to prevent it from being a problem. Drywall isn't as durable as plaster, so it can't be left unpainted.

The other big difference between plaster and drywall is in how they are finished. With plaster, there's a thin coating over the entire surface of the blueboard. With drywall, a coating of *drywall joint compound* (often called mud) is applied over paper tape at all the seams and at nail heads—not over the entire surface. The joint compound typically contains a variety of ingredients, such as the minerals gypsum, lime, talc, etc., plus additives such as antifreeze, preservatives, fungicides, and adhesives. These additives can outgas into the living space more than plaster.

We've found while plaster is theoretically more inert, sensitive people often tolerate drywall just fine—if they take a few precautions. First of all, because drywall must be painted, you must use a low-tox paint (#93). Second, you should use a low-tox joint compound. The healthiest one we've found is the M-100 Hi-Po Compound, made by Murco Wall Products (300 NE 21st St., Ft. Worth, TX 76106, 800-446-7124). It must be ordered from Texas, and is sold in powdered form, so it has be mixed with water on the job. (After the initial mixing, it should set for a while, then remixed to remove any lumps.) Because it contains no preservatives, don't mix more than you'll use in a day or it'll go bad. Once the compound is on the wall and completely dried, most contractors sand it smooth. If you're concerned about creating sanding dust, it can be smoothed with a damp sponge instead. Murco's product can also be used for texturing ceilings.

One last note on drywall: The sheets of drywall from different manufacturers are very similar in composition. So, one brand really isn't any healthier than another.

90. Why do you use foil-backed drywall in the houses you've built?

Foil-backed drywall is just like standard drywall—except that the backside is covered with a thin layer of aluminum foil. While it's often not kept in stock, it can usually be ordered from any dealer who sells standard drywall. We use it because the foil acts as a diffusion retarder.

We talked earlier (#38) about diffusion being insignificant at allowing air or pollutants to travel through solid surfaces. Well, diffusion is insignificant, but it's also very easy to deal with—so we do. Metals are quite good at retarding diffusion. So, by using foil-backed drywall that's sealed in an airtight manner, we're stopping both air movement and retarding diffusion.

We think foil-backed drywall is easy to use, but some builders prefer to use polyethylene sheeting inside the wall. It does basically the same thing, and it's only slightly less effective as a diffusion retarder than aluminum foil.

91. Should we be concerned about lead paint?

It depends on how old your house is. While the use of lead in paint started to decline about 1950, it wasn't banned in household paint until 1978. Lead is definitely a pollutant to be concerned about. But, it usually isn't a problem unless it's deteriorating, or disturbed during remodeling. So, if your house was built after 1978, and it's in good shape, there's a good chance that it doesn't have a lead paint problem. But, you may want to perform a simple test to make sure. You can buy inexpensive lead-testing kits at many hardware stores.

When it comes to lead—and many other pollutants for that matter—children are at more risk than adults, and children can be natural explorers. So, just because your house is lead paint-free, doesn't mean your kids are risk-free. They could be exposed to lead at a friend's house, or outdoors playing near an abandoned gas-station or battery-processing site. So, it can be a good idea for all children to have their blood tested for lead. If you suspect you have a problem, contact your local or state board of health, or call the EPA's National Lead Information Center at 800-532-3394 for guidance.

92. Can you recommend a healthy spackling compound?

Most typical spackling products have several additives, and they can be odorous. However, if you're just going to fill a few nail holes, you certainly won't be using much material. Therefore, a conventional spackling compound probably isn't going to be a serious outgassing source. For bigger jobs, or if you want to use as safe a product as possible, we recommend the M-100 Hi-Po Compound mentioned above (#89). It works for small jobs as well as large ones. If you're trying to cover up large cracks, you may want to use some tape (paper or fiberglass-mesh) along with the compound to reinforce it, in order to prevent the cracks from reappearing.

93. What paint should I get for my interior walls?

This is one of our most asked questions, and it's an important one. There are hundreds—sometimes thousands—of square feet of walls and ceilings in a house. If they're all painted, that can be a lot of surface area to which you and your family will be exposed. All paints outgas something when they're wet. Depending on the product, and depending on your degree of sensitivity, the outgassed chemicals could cause a variety of negative health effects.

Some products are definitely stronger than others when they're applied. And, some take a long time to outgas completely after they're dry. In general, we prefer water-based paints (and stains and clear finishes) because they outgas less initially, and the outgassing doesn't last too long. Solvent-based oil paints, on the other hand, are much stronger, and they can take weeks or months until they're completely cured. They often contain 40-60% solvent, and solvents are nasty chemicals. They often cause symptoms such as dizziness, nausea, and fatigue, and professional painters are more likely to get lung cancer, bladder cancer, and testicular cancer.

Most water-based paints contain a small amount of solvent—usually less than 5%. If you're not particularly sensitive, any water-based paint will probably be a reasonably good choice. To minimize your exposure, we recommend painting in mild weather when the windows can be left open. You can further reduce your exposure by using one or two window fans. If you want to use a healthier-than-average water-based paint, several major manufacturers (Benjamin Moore, Glidden, Kurfees, and Sherwin-Williams) have introduced zero-solvent (zero-VOC) paints. We still like to apply them with open windows, but they're very-low odor products, and they're often well tolerated by sensitive people.

Some very sensitive people have a great deal of trouble finding a tolerable paint. Fortunately, there are several paint companies who make alternative products that are even healthier than the zero-solvent paints distributed nationally. If you want to use one of these paints, you'll need to plan ahead because they must all be ordered through the mail. Each manufacturer has a slightly different concept as to what makes a paint healthier. For example, some use all-natural materials (#96), others use synthetic ingredients that outgas very little, and some make paint without preservatives or biocides. We can't say any one approach is better than another—they're just different—and none is universally tolerable for all sensitive people. That's why we recommend that sensitive individuals test several paints for personal tolerance (#15)—to see which one is best for them. To get you started, we've found that the alternative paints made by Best Paint Co. (5205 Ballard Ave. NW, Seattle, WA 98107, 206-783-9938) and Chem Safe Products (P.O. Box 33023, San Antonio, TX 78265, 210-657-5321) are tolerated fairly regularly by sensitive individuals.

94. Is there a healthy interior primer I can use?

Health-wise, water-based primers aren't a great deal different than water-based paints. But, occasionally we've had sensitive people tell us they tested a primer, then tested a paint, and both were tolerable. Then they primed and painted their walls, and were bothered by them. While this isn't common, it probably involves some kind of reaction between the two different coatings. This situation can be avoided by skipping the primer and simply applying an extra coat of paint.

95. How can I cover a water stain on my ceiling?

This is a case where you must use a specific type of product. That's because stains can bleed through most water-based paints. What you need is a special stain-blocking primer. There are several on the market. What we generally use is a product called B.I.N. It's an alcohol-based primer that contains shellac, and it's widely available. While the alcohol is very odorous, with plenty of ventilation it usually outgases quickly. You really only need to use a stain-blocking primer over the stain itself—you don't need to prime the entire ceiling. Once the stain has been primed, you can simply paint the ceiling with one of the products discussed above (#93). (Note: in some cases, an alcohol-based primer will react negatively with the Murco joint compound mentioned in #89.)

96. I have a latex allergy. Is there a healthy paint without latex?

Most water-based paints are called latex paints. However, that doesn't mean they all contain latex. In the paint industry, the work *latex* has come to simply mean *water-based*. In fact, many latex paints contain no latex at all but acrylic, vinyl, or some other resin instead. So, you may tolerate them just fine.

There's a specially made product that may interest you. It's a paint made with casein, which is a milk derivative. Manufactured by the Old Fashioned Milk Paint Co. (P.O. Box 222, Groton, MA 01450, 508-448-6336), it's a powdered material that must be mixed with water. While it's one of the healthiest paints available, it can have a slight milky odor that might bother someone with milk allergies. And, it has other drawbacks—it can be expensive, it doesn't cover very well, and it can get moldy in damp locations.

97. Is wallpaper a healthy product?

Today, many wallpapers are made of vinyl or have vinyl coatings, and they can definitely outgas into the living space. Another concern we have is with the glues and pastes used to attach them to the walls. Many contain fungicides so they won't get moldy. Some fungicides can negatively affect people as well as microbes.

Although we're not aware of any wallpapers that are healthier than others, we do have a few suggestions. First of all, you can unroll the wallpaper in an uncontaminated garage or in a well-ventilated, unused room to air out until it seems to have lost all its odor. For a paste, consider making your own with white flour and water. To minimize mold problems, you can add about a tablespoon of boric acid powder (usually sold in pharmacies) to each quart of paste.

You might also consider using less wallpaper to reduce your exposure. For example, using a narrow border around a room means less wallpaper, less paste, and less outgassing—plus, less expense.

98. Why is wall paneling unhealthy?

Four-by-eight-foot sheets of wall paneling are made with manufactured wood products that typically contain a potent urea-formaldehyde glue. There aren't any of these products that are perfect, but those made of hardboard (such as Masonite) are probably the least offensive because they use the least amount of glue.

Personally, our preference is for solid-wood paneling. It can be more expensive, but it contains no formaldehyde-based glue. If you can tolerate soft-woods, pine paneling can be reasonably priced. But, there are low-cost hardwoods, too, such as tulip poplar.

If solid-wood paneling looks like it's going to be too expensive to use in an entire room, you can get a very nice effect by just covering the lower third of the walls with wainscoting. In many cases, a simple horizontal chair rail can dress up a wall at even less cost.

XII.
Interior floors

XII.

99. Why don't you like wall-to-wall carpeting?

As we said earlier (#11), we consider carpeting to be one of the most common polluters in homes. Most carpeting is made of chemically treated, chemically dyed, synthetic fibers attached to a synthetic backing with a synthetic glue. It's then installed over synthetic padding—sometimes with another synthetic glue. It isn't unusual for all these materials to outgas over a hundred different chemicals into the air. It's been shown that, in some cases, the outgassing from carpeting can be truly dangerous. In laboratory experiments, mice exposed to some carpet samples have suffered severe neurological symptoms and some actually died.

Another problem with carpet is that it's a perfect home to microorganisms such as mold, mildew, and dust mites. It isn't unusual for there to be tens-of-millions of tiny microbes in every square foot of carpeting. It's also a reservoir for everything you track indoors on your shoes—soil, lawn chemicals, lead dust from chalking house paint, asbestos fibers from automotive brake linings, animal feces, and anything else found on the ground outdoors.

Wall-to-wall carpeting is virtually impossible to clean thoroughly, so it's always going to be a source of allergens. Plus, cleaning can cause additional problems. Routine vacuuming often stirs up dust—making it airborne. Damp-cleaning processes can add enough moisture to cause the microorganisms living in the carpet to thrive. Plus, most carpet shampoos contain fragrance, solvents, or other chemicals that can bother some people.

100. I know it's unhealthy, but I still want carpet. What's the best kind to buy?

The best advice we can give is to look for a product with as little odor as possible. It'll help to take someone along with you who has a good sense of smell when you go shopping for carpet and padding. This is imperfect advice because some of the chemicals outgassed don't have an odor. If you can't find a low-odor carpet, you can roll it out in an uncontaminated garage and let it air out there before you bring it indoors for installation. Furthermore, you should install the carpet with tack strips rather than an adhesive.

Many people believe natural-fiber carpets are inherently healthier. Sometimes they are, but that's not always the case. Natural fibers are often chemically dyed or treated and wool carpet is routinely treated with mothproofing chemicals. Actually, some 100%-nylon carpets are less bothersome than some natural carpets. Whatever kind of carpet you choose, we highly recommend using a central vacuum cleaner to maintain it (#133).

Area rugs can have several advantages over carpet. First of all, you can often find them locally made of cotton or other natural fibers at reasonable prices. Some may even been dyed using natural plant dyes. If they have any odor when new, they can usually be laundered in a washing machine or hung outdoors until odor-free. As a result, they're much easier to keep clean than wall-to-wall carpet. If a larger area rug won't fit in your washing machine, you can take it outdoors and beat it over a line—but be sure and wear a good dust mask.

101. Wood floors are always a healthy flooring choice, right?

Almost any hard-surfaced floor is healthier and easier to keep clean than carpeting. Traditionally, wood floors were made of tongue-and-groove boards that were individually nailed down, sanded in place, then finished. These were often low-tox floors—as long as low-tox finishes were used. Today, some wood flooring is made in a sandwich—like plywood—and held together with a glue. It's often attached to the floor with another glue. Many products are now prefinished using a variety of different materials. We prefer solid wood.

For very sensitive people the choice of wood is important. That's because they may react to one type of wood but not to another. Oak is the most common wood-flooring material, but it can have a strong natural odor. Many sensitive individuals can tolerate oak—once it's been finished. For those who can't, maple, beech, birch, or another hardwood may be a better choice. If you aren't bothered by softwoods, a yellow-pine floor can be an attractive, less expensive option.

102. Does my contractor have to use asphalt-impregnated felt paper under my new hardwood floor?

He really doesn't have to use anything under the new floor. But, the felt paper sometimes helps minimize squeaks. In older homes having a subfloor made of square-edged boards, the felt paper also helps prevent dust from moving between the individual boards. If asphalt-impregnated felt paper is used, it'll be underneath the finish floor, so it won't be directly exposed to the living space. As a result, the outgassing won't be serious. But just to be safe, we don't use it. Instead, we usually use builder's foil (#33). We get it in 3'-wide rolls made of Kraft paper with aluminum foil on both sides.

103. What's the healthiest finish for hardwood floors?

Selecting a low-tox finish is actually the most important health decision with wood flooring. Over the years, shellac, acrylic, urea-formaldehyde, and other resins have been used in floor finishes. More recently, *water-based urethane* finishes have become popular. They're durable and easy-to-maintain, and they outgas quickly. We often talk to sensitive people who tolerate them less than a week after application. You should stay away from *oil-based* urethanes because they often take months to outgas completely. Many of the manufacturers of prefinished flooring are now using the newer water-based urethanes.

Personally, we don't like to stain wood floors. We like the natural color variation of the wood. But if you want a stain, simply choose a water-based version that doesn't have much odor. Some are quite strong, but the milder ones will usually be sealed in by the water-based urethane finish. If you're very sensitive, you'll probably want to have a sample of flooring that's been stained and finished to test for personal tolerance. (#15)

By the way, water-based urethane finishes can be used in many different applications. We use them on furniture, cabinets, interior doors, and trim.

104. Is linoleum a healthy flooring option?

Real linoleum is made with linseed oil, pine resins, powdered wood, and pigments on a jute backing. It's an attractive and natural product, but it has a fairly strong odor when new. So, it's not always tolerated by sensitive people. Because it's subject to water damage, it must be coated with a sealant (which can also be bothersome) to protect it, and it isn't a good idea to use it in very wet areas like bathrooms. Linoleum must be attached to the floor with an adhesive (use a water-based version!), but in the right situation, it can be a durable and long-lasting floor covering.

105. Can vinyl be a good flooring choice?

Vinyl flooring can also have a strong odor when new. But, some sensitive people have had good luck rolling it out in an uncontaminated garage—or in a well-ventilated, unused room—until it airs out before installing it. Vinyl is more resistant to water than linoleum, so it can be used in damp areas.

Vinyl is usually available in wider widths than linoleum. That means it can sometimes be installed without an adhesive. For example, if a room is less than 12' wide (the usual width of a roll of vinyl), you can remove the baseboard trim, cut the vinyl carefully to fit, then reinstall the baseboard on top of it to hold it in place. You'll need to use a thin wood or aluminum threshold at the doors. As an alternative, self-stick vinyl tiles have an adhesive that's sometimes not too odorous.

106. I'd like to use ceramic tile for my floors, but isn't it expensive?

There's actually a wide range of prices for ceramic tile. Some discount building centers have very good prices on glazed floor tiles, and some tile companies sell slightly imperfect tiles (seconds) at a discount. Seconds often have minor color imperfections or tiny chips on an edge that can only be seen if you get down on your knees and look carefully. But, ceramic tile can still be costly because of the labor involved. If you're handy, and regularly take on home-repair projects, you can save a great deal of money by installing ceramic tile yourself. The few simple tools you'll need (nippers, tile cutter, trowel, and grout squeegee) can either be purchased or rented. John's *Healthy House Building* book shows how to install a healthy tile floor in a step-by-step manner.

We like ceramic-tile floors a lot. We think they're one of the healthiest, most attractive options available. If you plan to live in your house for some time, you should realize that they're also very long lasting. You'll have to replace vinyl several times before a ceramic-tile floor is worn out. So, in the long run, ceramic tile can be very cost effective.

107. Aren't ceramic-tile floors uncomfortable to stand on?

Some people don't like ceramic-tile (or concrete) floors because they feel they are tiring to stand on. However, you can save your feet by placing soft natural-fiber area rugs wherever you spend a lot of time standing—such as in front of the kitchen or bathroom sink, stove, etc.

Ceramic-tile floors are often cool to the touch. In warm weather, they can feel refreshing to bare feet. However, in cold climates, they can be too cold for some people. So, it pays to have a well-insulated floor. Again, natural-fiber area rugs strategically placed around the house can improve your comfort level—or you may simply be happy wearing slippers in the winter. Some ceramic-tile floors are radiantly heated, making they very warm and comfortable when it's cold outdoors.

108. My house isn't built on a concrete slab. Can I still have ceramic-tile floors?

Yes you can, but if you want to install ceramic tile over a wood or plywood subfloor, you should first make sure the floor is stiff enough. If it flexes too much, you'll end up with cracked tile. One of the best ways to install tile on a wooden subfloor is to first put down a layer of *cementitious board* (Durock is widely available, but there are other comparable brands). For a long-lasting installation, the cementitious board is attached to the subfloor with thinset mortar (#109) and plenty of screws. Then, the tile is installed on top of that with some more thinset mortar. Once the mortar has cured, you're ready for grout.

Cementitious boards are made of Portland cement and a few other ingredients. They're usually $1/2$" thick, and they can have a slight odor. However, once installed, the odor is rarely noticeable because it's under the tile. Once the tile is in place, the whole assembly functions as a fairly good diffusion retarder (#38). So, if the subfloor is made of plywood, it usually can't outgas through the tile into the living space.

109. Are there low-odor mortars and grouts that can be used with ceramic tile?

We've found that most thinset mortars are relatively low-odor products that are made with Portland cement and a few additives. But, occasionally, we'll come across a brand that has a very strong chemical odor. In one case, someone sent us a sample of a product that had a very nasty odor. It was the same brand that we'd just used on a project, and ours didn't have any odor at all. Yet, they were being sold as identical products. As it turns out, they were made in different factories, and the suppliers of the additives were different companies. Still, most of these products generally don't have much odor, and once they're covered with tile, they're usually just fine. If you get a sample before you start a project, mix it with water and sniff it to determine if there's any odor. The "bad stuff" has a very strong, synthetic-chemical odor.

Because grout is directly exposed to the living space, we usually make our own in order to avoid additives completely. For typical $1/4$" joints, mix 2 parts clean, dry sand with 1 part Portland cement, then add water. Apply it like any other grout. If you want a colored grout, you can add the same natural-mineral pigments that bricklayers use in their mortar.

Many of the additives in ready-mixed grouts cause them to cure slowly. So, if you have no additives, you'll need to do something called *damp curing*. That means, when you're finished grouting, you'll need to cover the floor with a sheet of plastic for 72 hours. That'll help the grout retain moisture, causing it to cure slowly. A few commercially-made grouts also require damp curing. They have the fewest additives, and are usually healthy choices.

110. Don't ceramic-tile floors need to be sealed?

Yes and no. Unglazed tiles can, indeed, get dirty. That's why they're usually sealed. To avoid sealers (some sealers are better than others), we prefer glazed tiles because the glass-like surface is durable, long-lasting, stain resistant, and easy-to-keep-clean. Most of the time, all you need is a damp mop to keep a glazed-tile floor looking good.

The grout between the tiles can also get dirty. It's more absorbent and more easily stained than glazed tile. We've found that darker grouts hide stains easier than light-colored grouts. We've also found an easy way to remove many common stains from grout using *Fullers earth* —a dry, powdered, natural clay you can usually order through a pharmacy. Mix a little Fuller's earth and water to make a paste, apply it to the stain, and allow it to set overnight. In the morning, you can brush it off with a stiff broom, then vacuum it up.

There's one type of sealant that works well on grout. It's a low-tox product made of sodium silicate, which is also called *water glass*. When it's applied to grout, it reacts with the calcium in the cement and forms a crystalline structure in the surface of the grout. It can be time consuming to apply—you need to use an artist's brush—but it can be very long lasting. Brand names include Penetrating Water Stop (AFM Enterprises, Inc., 350 W. Ash St. #700, San Diego, CA 92101, 619-239-0321) and Penetrating Sealer (Aqua Mix, 9419 Ann St., Santa Fe Springs, CA 90670, 800-366-6877).

XIII.
Cabinets,
doors, and
trim

XIII.

111. How healthy are most kitchen cabinets?

As a rule, the majority of new cabinets—kitchen, bath, etc.—are quite unhealthy. This is because manufacturers all use man-made wood products—hardboard, particle board, and plywood—which contain a potent urea-formaldehyde glue. Even expensive cabinets are made with these materials, and they outgas formaldehyde for years (#10). Although the doors and drawer fronts may be made of solid wood, the end panels, backs, shelves, drawer bottoms, and drawer sides are made of noxious wood products. They can have an attractive thin wood veneer on the surface, but it does little to block formaldehyde. Some manufacturers claim they make their cabinets out of "solid wood," but they're playing games with definitions. If you ask if they use plywood, they'll answer, "Yes, that plywood is solid wood."

When man-made wood products have a plastic or vinyl surfacing, it can block some of the emissions, but almost never enough for sensitive people to tolerate new cabinets. This is because in commercially made cabinets, the plastic or vinyl surfacing rarely covers all the edges, and it often has holes drilled in it for shelf supports.

While the cabinet materials are bad enough, the clear finishes used are often worse. Most manufactures use a urea-formaldehyde clear finish that is one of the strongest formaldehyde emitters found in houses. The good news is that it's so powerful, it's usually done outgassing after 4-6 months. After that, you've still got the formaldehyde in the plywood, particle board, and hardboard to contend with.

112. Can't I just coat problem cabinets with a sealant to make them safe?

To be effective, a sealant must be applied to all surfaces—top, bottom, front, back, sides, edges, and all nooks and crannies. We've talked to a number of sensitive people who have done this and they almost always say the same thing: "It was a lot of work. We put 4 coats of sealant on everything, and it did help—but it didn't help enough." You get imperfect results because most sealers are imperfect at blocking emissions.

Benjamin Moore Paint Co. has a sealer called Impervo that was tested in Canada and found to block 100% of formaldehyde emissions, but it's an oil-based paint. For sensitive people, it probably wouldn't be any more tolerable than the formaldehyde. Plus, it won't do much for the appearance of your attractive new oak cabinets to slap a few coats of paint on them.

113. What healthy options do I have if I want new wood cabinets?

Currently Neff Kitchen Manufacturers Ltd. (6 Melanie Dr., Brampton, ON Canada L6T 4K9, 905-791-7770) is the only company making cabinets available nationally with reduced levels of formaldehyde. They still use plywood, but their raw materials use less urea-formaldehyde glue than most other cabinet-grade products. These cabinets are better-than-average, but they're probably not healthy enough for sensitive people.

One of the healthiest options is to have cabinets custom made with solid wood throughout. Although most cabinet shops don't routinely do this, many have the ability to do so. We've used this option several times, and have learned a few tricks to make construction easier and a bit less expensive. For example, you can use a less-expensive wood for the shelves and insides, and just use the more costly oak or walnut for the exposed fronts. We also have eliminated the back panels. So, when you look into our cabinets, you just see the painted kitchen (or bathroom) wall. For drawer bottoms, we use galvanized (zinc coated) sheet metal. It's easy to clean, and easy to substitute for a more-expensive solid-wood panel. For the wide shelves in base cabinets, we've also used galvanized sheet metal. We just measure what we need and have a local sheet-metal shop fold up pieces with mounting flanges, and then screw them to solid-wood end panels. You can also substitute glass for upper cabinet shelves, or for the panels in upper cabinet door fronts.

Some people have made the cabinet shelves and end panels out of construction-grade plywood because it's made with a much-less-potent phenol-formaldehyde glue. A product called Medex (Medite Corporation, P.O. Box 4040, Medford, OR 97501, 800-676-3339) is also sometimes used because it contains a formaldehyde-free glue. These are great options—if you aren't particularly sensitive. But, we know of sensitive people who are bothered by these materials because of their natural pine odor. They can sometimes be made tolerable by covering all surfaces with a hard plastic laminate (such as Formica). This can give you an attractive European look.

We've also heard of people buying cheap metal cabinets, ripping the fronts off, and attaching attractive new fronts made of solid wood. With a little ingenuity, you can have healthy cabinets—it just takes a little thought and preplanning.

114. I'm having trouble finding metal cabinets. Are they still being made?

They certainly are, although there aren't a lot of suppliers. You can still buy the plain, white cabinets that were common in the 1950s, or you can buy attractive textured-metal cabinets in a variety of designer colors. You can even get cabinets made completely of low-tox stainless steel.

The least-toxic finish on painted cabinets is usually a powder coating. It consists of a special powdered paint that's sprayed onto hot metal and baked on. If you're interested in metal cabinets, ask about soundproofing materials. Some manufactures use fiberboard or some other material inside hollow doors, but they'll often leave it out on special request. Suppliers of metal cabinets include Davis Kitchens (P.O. Box D, New Buffalo, MI 49117, 800-553-2847), Fillip Metal Cabinet Co. (701 N. Albany St., Chicago, IL 60612, 773-826-7373), and Kitchens and Baths by Don Johnson (Merchandise Mart #1375, Chicago, IL 60654, 773-548-2436).

115. Are plastic countertops healthy?

Some are, some aren't. If you look underneath those made with a high-pressure plastic laminate (such as Formica), you'll invariably see unfinished particle board—which is outgassing formaldehyde downward. If you're having new countertops made, there are a couple of things you can do to reduce emissions. First, you can substitute construction-grade plywood or Medex (#113) for the particle board. You can also cover all surfaces—not just the top and exposed edges— with plastic laminate. The plastic itself is hard enough that it doesn't outgas much, and it's dense enough that it's fairly good at blocking emissions. You can also specify that a water-based contact adhesive be used—rather than the usual solvent-based version—but this isn't critical if all surfaces are covered with plastic laminate.

Corian, which is made by DuPont, is one of several solid-surfacing materials now on the market. They're all synthetic products, made with acrylic or polyester resin and marble dust. Most are fairly inert, and they're often well tolerated by sensitive people.

However, sometimes, to save money, these countertops are made with a solid-surfacing material laminated on top of a plywood or particleboard base, which can outgas formaldehyde. For the healthiest installation, you should just use the solid-surfacing material itself. To be sturdy enough, the countertops may need to be made with a thicker material, or have stiffeners attached to the bottom.

116. Why do you like stainless steel for kitchen countertops?

Stainless steel is the healthiest countertop option available. It's been used for decades in hospitals, commercial kitchens, and laboratories. Stainless can withstand hot pots and it won't support microbial growth. Neither will it stain, crack, nor chip. In addition, it doesn't require a sealant, and it never needs polish or wax. We've put several stainless-steel countertops into healthy houses, and they earn high marks from homeowners because they're so easy to keep clean and so great to work on.

Sometimes, a thin gauge of stainless is laminated to a plywood base material. We've always used 14-gauge stainless, which is stiff enough that it doesn't need a base. These countertops are always custom made, and measurements must be precise because stainless countertops can't easily be trimmed to fit. We've had them made with the countertop and backsplash in one seamless piece. For a sink, there are two choices. While it can be costly, you can have the sink welded into the countertop with all seams polished until they're invisible. Or, you can just use a standard drop-in sink. To locate a fabricator, look in your phone book under Commercial Kitchen Suppliers. Most major cites will have one or more companies listed that regularly provide stainless-steel countertops.

117. I'm chemically sensitive. What kind of wood trim should I use in my new house?

It depends on just how sensitive you are. For most people, trim made of solid pine is a very good choice, but some sensitive people are bothered by its natural aroma. If your sensitivities aren't severe, you may be able to tolerate pine just fine once it's finished. We like to use the clear water-based urethane finishes that are often used on floors (#103). If pine is a problem for you, trim made of hardwood (such as oak, maple, or poplar) is often available in many parts of the country. In the Midwest, we routinely use tulip-poplar for trim because it's quite attractive. And, because it grows here, it's cheaper than pine.

118. What kind of interior doors are healthiest?

Doors can be made from a variety of materials: solid wood, plywood, particle board, plastic, resin-impregnated paper, etc. Those made completely of solid wood are definitely the healthiest. Most lumber yards and building-supply centers can readily supply solid-wood doors made of pine, and they can usually order them made with hardwoods such as oak or poplar. In addition, there are custom cabinet shops in most parts of the country that can supply solid-wood doors in a variety of styles.

Steel doors can also be used, but they tend to look rather institutional. Some interior steel doors have soundproofing materials or stiffeners inside, but the steel skin usually prevents most of the odors from escaping. Metal doors can be taken to an automotive body shop to be painted in an attractive color (#44). For closets, companies such as Slimfold Products (868 Murray Rd., Dothan, AL 36303, 800-633-7553) offer pre-finished metal bi-fold closet doors with louvers or embossed panels, or mirrored by-pass doors that are healthy options.

XIV.
Furnishing a
healthy house

XIV.

119. We're getting ready to move into our new healthy house. Do you have any additional advice?

Congratulations! By using healthy building materials and installing a ventilation system, you now have a healthy structure. However, you must realize that what you put inside your house is just as important as how you built it. We've heard of cases where healthy houses were filled with unhealthy furnishings and maintained with unhealthy cleaning products. The result was poor indoor air quality. Fortunately, there are plenty of healthy products out there that can be substituted for all the unhealthy ones. Lynn's book, *The Healthy Household*, goes into interiors in considerable depth, but the following questions and answers cover the highlights.

120. Antique furniture was made before particleboard and other synthetic materials became popular, so it's healthy, right?

Not necessarily, old furniture can be contaminated with musty smells, tobacco smoke, pesticides, and perfume odors—all things that affect air quality. Some pieces are actually moldy. If an antique piece has been refinished recently, it may be bothersome because of a noxious stripper that was used, or because of an oil-based stain or finish.

We have an antique oak desk that belonged to John's great grandmother. Over the years it picked up a wide variety of odors, and it was too bothersome to bring it into our healthy house. We thought about stripping the finish off ourselves (3M has a low-tox product that's widely available called Safest Stripper), but decided to take it to a commercial stripper. They had more powerful stripping chemicals, the correct safety equipment, and they knew where to properly dispose of the spent stripper and old finish. Once it was stripped, it didn't have the original odors, but it did smell of stripper. So, we put it in the garage and let it air out for a couple of months. Once it was aired out, we finished it with a water-based urethane floor finish (#103). It's now odor free and sitting in our entry hall.

121. I think outgassing from some of my new upholstered furniture is affecting my health. Any suggestions?

This can be due to outgassing from materials used in the framework, artificial stuffing, synthetic fabrics, dyes, or stain-resistant treatments. It can be a difficult situation, and your options are limited—but there are options. The first option is to keep the furniture in the house. This is only viable if you aren't seriously affected, and it's possible for you to avoid spending very much time in the same room with it. If it's more-than-a-little bothersome, and it's brand new, you may try to get the store to take it back. Sometimes, new furniture just needs time to air out. We've known people who had to place a new couch in an uncontaminated garage, or on a covered patio, to air out naturally for as long as a year before they could tolerate it indoors. If you must keep a piece of furniture indoors, there's a very densely woven cotton fabric, called *barrier cloth*, that can be draped over it to block some of the outgassing. You can get barrier cloth through the mail from Janice Corp. (198 Route 46, Budd Lake, NJ 07828, 800-JANICES).

If your furniture is really bothersome, you may need to consider selling it or donating it to someone who is less sensitive than you are. Whatever, remember that your health is of primary importance. Don't worry what people will think if you don't have a couch in your living room. And, don't worry about money wasted. Money is less important than your physical well being.

122. We're in the market for a new couch. Does anyone make them with healthy materials?

Yes, there are some mail-order sources that offer upholstered furniture made with solid wood frames and all-natural stuffing and fabrics. A number of different styles are available. In some cases you can actually specify organically raised cotton.

Catalog suppliers of healthy furniture include Furnature (319 Washington St., Brighton, MA 02135, 617-782-3939) and The Natural Alternative (11577 124th St. N., Hugo, MN 55038, 612-351-7165). If you're handy with a sewing machine, you might look into a metal-framed patio couch, and make your own cushions out of healthy stuffing and fabric. Dona Designs (1611 Bent Tree St., Seagoville, TX 75159, 972-287-7834) sells organically raised cotton batting.

123. Do you think the extra cost of an all-natural mattress is worth the expense?

Absolutely. You spend about a third of your life in bed, so it should be as healthy as is possible. Most mattresses are made of synthetic materials, and they have various chemical coatings and treatments. For example, Federal law requires that mattresses be treated with flame retardants.

Healthy mattresses can be made of all-cotton or wool. If your doctor feels it's a good idea, he can actually write you a prescription for a mattress without flame retardants. Suppliers include Janice Corp. (198 Route 46, Budd Lake, NJ 07828, 800-JANICES) and Nontoxic Environments, Inc., P.O. Box 384, New Market, NH 03857, 800-789-4348). If there's a mattress manufacturer in your town, Dona Designs (1611 Bent Tree St., Seagoville, TX 75159, 972-287-7834) can sell you the organic cotton padding and the covering fabrics so they can make a mattress to your exact specifications.

124. I don't like the appearance of metal mini-blinds. Why do you use them for your windows?

Everyone's taste is different. We happen to like metal mini-blinds because they come in a wide range of colors, slat widths, and styles. Once you've let the new paint air out for a while, they're quite inert. They won't deteriorate like fabric curtains do in the sun, and they can be adjusted to provide just the amount of privacy or sunlight you desire. In addition, they're easy to clean with a vacuum, and they're affordable.

125. I'm very chemically sensitive and need a new stove. What do you suggest I get?

This is another one of our most asked questions. First of all, you should avoid gas ranges. We feel the negative health effects associated with combustion by-products are just too serious for them to be a consideration (#65). As far as electric stoves are concerned, the bad news is that there aren't any that are perfect. They can all have an odor from the new heating elements, warm plastic jacketing on wiring, outgassing from insulation, or odors from oven coatings.

We have a fairly new electric stove in our house, and it's very healthy. However, it wasn't that way when we bought it. Based on past experience, we knew that Lynn would be bothered by conventional spiral heating elements. So, we decided to get a model with a smooth glass top having burners hidden just under the surface. We opted for a self-cleaning model. When we first turned it on, it smelled quite strongly. The manufacturer said it was normal and the odor would eventually go away, but it seemed like it was going to take a long time.

We have a 220-volt outlet in our garage, so we put the new stove in the garage and plugged it in there. Then we turned it on. The top aired out fairly quickly, but the oven had a stronger odor. So, we activated the oven's self cleaning cycle—which operates at a higher-than-normal temperature. Over a couple of weeks, we ran the cleaning cycle twice a day—about 30 times in all. This was enough heat to bake out all the synthetic odors. Today the stove is indoors and is just fine.

126. I've heard of something called a safe haven. Just what is that?

When someone first learns that they're chemically sensitive, it can be discouraging to hear that their house—and everything in it—could be contributing to their ill health. Very few of us can afford to build a new house and completely furnish it overnight with healthy materials. What often helps (in some cases, it helps a lot) is to create one room in a house that's as healthy as possible. If good air quality can be maintained in, say, a bedroom, a sensitive person can often regain a certain level of their health back by spending eight hours or more in that room every day. This safe haven is also sometimes called an oasis or sanctuary because it provides relief from an otherwise continuous exposure to air pollutants.

To create a safe haven, you'll first need to remove everything from the bedroom. Then, the walls will need to be thoroughly cleaned with a tolerable, low-odor cleaner. If the clean, empty room is still bothersome, it's sometimes necessary to seal off the heating/cooling registers to prevent air from entering from other parts of the house. If you suspect the flooring or the paint on the walls to be a problem, they can be covered with builders foil (#33) to seal in any outgassing. Once the room itself is tolerable, you can bring in (one at time) different pieces of furniture to see how you react to them. You should only have items in the safe haven that are perfectly tolerable.

You should be aware that a safe haven is often not a cure-all. But it can be a significant step toward improved health. For in-depth instructions on how to create a safe haven, check out Lynn's book, *The Healthy Household.*

XV.
Maintaining a healthy house

XV.

127. I can't tolerate the artificial fragrances in laundry products. Are there any healthier options?

There are a number of mail-order companies that sell fragrance-free products, and they're also often available at health-food stores or co-op groceries. Catalog suppliers include N.E.E.D.S. (527 Charles Ave. #12-A, Syracuse, NY 13209, 800-634-1380) and Nontoxic Environments, Inc. (P.O. Box 384, New Market, NH 03857, 800-789-4348).

If you live in or near a large city, look in the telephone directory under Chemical Suppliers. There should be companies listed that sell all kinds of nasty industrial chemicals. However, they also often sell unscented borax, or unscented washing soda (sometimes called sal soda, or sodium sesquicarbonate)—both of which can be used in the laundry. You may need to purchase 50-100# bags, but buying in bulk is considerably cheaper per pound than buying in small quantities. Sometimes, adding a cup of white vinegar to the wash water can help remove odors.

You may run into another problem with artificial fragrances if you're shopping for a new washer or dryer. That's because many manufacturers put scented samples of detergent or fabric softener inside new machines at the factory. If you can't get a company to ship an appliance without free samples, your best solution is to remove the offending products from the washer or dryer immediately. Then, run the washer (without clothes) several times with unscented borax, baking soda, or white vinegar until the odor dissipates. Likewise, run the empty dryer on its highest temperature setting until all the perfume odors are gone. If your utility room has a window, keep it open during the entire "decontamination" period.

128. How important is it to use unscented cleaning products and cosmetics, and natural-fiber clothing?

Scents and perfumes very often trigger reactions in chemically sensitive people and they bother many individuals with conventional allergies. We feel it's very important to use unscented products throughout your home. Because fragrances are formulated to spread and cling, they can quickly saturate an entire house and be difficult to remove.

Scented cosmetics can be especially problematic for sensitive people because they're applied directly to the skin. Your clothing is also in direct contact with your skin. We've found that untreated natural-fiber clothing (cotton, wool, linen, ramie, hemp, etc.) is a good option because it outgases no synthetic odors. And, we choose only those items that can be easily cleaned at home with unscented laundry products.

129. The house we just moved into smells perfumy. What can I do to remove the odor?

This is a difficult problem, with no really good answer. Unfortunately, perfume, potpourri, incense, and other natural or artificial fragrances can saturate walls, floors, cabinets, etc. and be extremely difficult to remove completely.

Washing walls (and ceilings) with TSP (tri-sodium phosphate), which is available at many paint and hardware stores, can often help. Opening the windows and blowing plenty of air through the house with window fans for an extended period of time seems to help as much as anything.

Sometimes, repainting will seal in the fragrance odor. But, if the smell is really strong, it can bleed through the new paint. Get a low-tox paint and try it in one room before repainting the whole house.

Sometimes, it's just the walls inside a closet that are saturated with fragrance. In that case, "wallpapering" the walls in a closet with builders foil (#33), or household aluminum foil, often helps.

130. Do you think a central vacuum is worth the added expense?

Yes, we do. There are two problems with conventional vacuum cleaners. Most have very inefficient filters, so the smallest dust particles travel right through them and get blown back into the room—often in your face. The exhaust can also stir up dust that hasn't been picked up yet.

There are a number of manufacturers who sell portable vacuums with very efficient filters. Some can be quite expensive, and even though the exhaust is highly filtered, it can still stir up room dust, causing it to become airborne.

Central vacuums usually cost more than typical portable vacuums, but they're often comparable in price to the more-efficient models. If their exhaust air is vented outdoors (as it is with most central vacuums), they're the healthiest type of vacuum to operate. They're also very convenient to use. You just plug a hose into special wall inlets placed strategically around your house. Hoses come in several lengths, so you can usually clean two or three rooms at a time before you need to plug into a different inlet.

131. I can't seem to get the dry-cleaning odors out of my clothes? What do you suggest I do?

This is another tough question, for which there's no good answer. Most dry-cleaners use a petroleum-based solvent, perchloroethylene (perc), as the cleaning agent. (In some cases, they also use soaps and detergents.) The perc odor can easily impregnate the fibers of your clothing.

Airing freshly dry-cleaned clothing is the only real solution. Hanging the clothes outdoors in a breeze seems to help the most. Unfortunately, for some sensitive individuals, no amount of airing is enough. For them, dry cleaning simply isn't an option, and they must stick with clothing they can launder at home.

132. How do I deal with mold?

The first thing you need to do is determine how the mold problem started. Mold and mildew grow where there's too much water or where there's high relative humidity. If you fix any water problems and lower the humidity, the mold will become dormant and stop growing. The next step is to clean everything thoroughly to remove as many dormant mold spores as possible. If everything remains dry and at a low humidity, a mold problem shouldn't return.

If mold has stained the walls, you may need to repaint to spruce things up. Don't expect paint alone to solve a mold problem. Mold needs moisture to live, and if you don't dry things out, it'll just start eating the new paint.

Often it isn't practical to try and kill the mold. That's because many fungicidal chemicals can be bothersome to people, too. Besides, allergic people react to dead mold as well as live mold because they're affected by certain proteins, and the proteins can be alive or dead and still trigger a allergic reaction. That's why clean-up is so important. Still, an unscented borax-and-water solution, or a 3%-hydrogen-peroxide solution (the concentration commonly sold in drug stores), both have some fungicidal properties. So, that's what we like to use when cleaning up moldy areas. These happen to be odor-free and relatively harmless to people.

133. What's a healthy way to combat sugar ants in my kitchen and clothing moths in my closet?

While ants can invade the cleanest of kitchens, you should first make sure there's nothing around for them to eat. A sticky spot of spilled orange juice on the floor can be a real treat to an ant.

The ants' nest is usually outdoors, but they send out scouts to look for food, and the scouts lay down scent trails for others to follow. You can often follow the trails and find where they're getting in, so you can caulk or seal up the entry points. Then, you should clean everything again to destroy the scent trails.

If you can't seem to keep them out, sprinkling talcum powder near the entry points and along trails often takes care of them. It works by clinging to their bodies and preventing normal respiration. Ants take air in through tiny holes (spiracles) in their bodies, and the talcum powder clogs the holes, so they suffocate and die.

Clothing moths like to eat the lanolin on wool. (Actually, it's moth larva that do the damage.) If woolens haven't been cleaned, they can contain human body oils and food particles that the larva also eat. Contrary to popular belief, cedar isn't a good moth repellent and mothballs (usually made of noxious chemicals) can be dangerous to humans and the environment.

To prevent moth damage in a healthy way, first clean your wool items before you store them. Then place them in tightly sealed bags or containers. A cedar chest prevents moth damage, not because it's cedar, but because it seals tightly. If moths can't get your woolens, they can't damage them. (Note: Cedar odors are often bothersome to sensitive people.)

Another way to prevent damage is to tumble your woolens in a clothes dryer for fifteen minutes once a month, or vigorously shake them out periodically. The moths eggs and larva are fragile and aren't firmly attached to the fibers, so they're easy to remove.

Afterword

We wrote this book to empower you—so you could understand what makes a house healthy. It's a sad state of affairs that a book like this is necessary. After all, as Americans we all spend 80-90% of our time indoors. So we should be able to assume that our indoor environments are hospitable. But, they aren't.

There's no need for our houses to continue making us sick. Healthy technology exists. It's just that unhealthy technology has become the unquestioned norm. What we need is to become aware of the healthy options available to us. That's where this book comes in. Here's to your healthy house.

About the authors

John Bower has a BS in Industrial Education from Purdue University and a MA in Education from Ball State University. He has been involved with healthy-house construction since 1984 as a designer, builder, consultant, writer, and lecturer. He has written scores of articles, and three books (*The Healthy House, Healthy House Building, and Understanding Ventilation*). John is the recipient of a Professional Achievement Award from *Professional Builder* magazine and is on the editorial advisory board of *Indoor Environment Review*.

Lynn Marie Bower has a BS in Education (magna cum laude) from Western Michigan University. She has taught school and is an accomplished artist. In the 1970s, she acquired multiple chemical sensitivity (MCS) as the result of an extensive home remodeling project. Since then, she has written dozens of articles, co-edited a stateside MCS-support-group newsletter, and authored *The Healthy Household*—all with a focus on achieving a healthy lifestyle.

Together, John and Lynn have written *The Healthy House Answer Book* and produced a video (*Your House, Your Health*). In 1992, they started The Healthy House Institute—an independent resource center offering books and videos containing practical information for designers, architects, contractors, and homeowners interested in making houses healthy.

Index

A

B

Notes

Notes

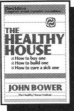
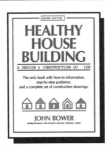

Available from The Healthy House Institute

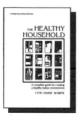

$17.95

The Healthy Household offers hundreds of practical suggestions for improving your indoor environment. With chapters devoted to cleaning products, personal-care items, clothing, linens, interior decorating, life-styles, housekeeping, air and water quality, and electromagnetic radiation, no other book matches its completeness. It is an essential reference for anyone interested in their family's health—especially those who are chemically sensitive. Trade paperback, 6" x 9", 480 pages.

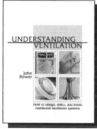

$31.95

Understanding Ventilation covers all aspects of exchanging the air in houses: infiltration, equipment selection, design, heat-recovery ventilators, sizing, costs, controls, whole-house filters, distribution, and possible problems that a ventilation system can cause—and all in easy-to-understand language. Any architect, builder, or homeowner interested in maintaining a healthy, comfortable indoor environment will find this manual indispensable. Fully illustrated. Hardcover, $8\frac{1}{2}$" x 11", 432 pages.

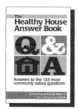

$8.95

The Healthy House Answer Book is a user-friendly construction and life-style reference guide you won't want to be without. Here are answers to all those questions you've been wondering about—as well as answers to other important questions you didn't even think to ask. Carpet, paints, cabinets, air and water filters, furnaces, plywood, laundry soap, and many more topics, are fully covered with concise, easy-to-understand explanations. Trade paperback, $5\frac{1}{4}$" x $8\frac{1}{4}$", 192 pages.

Order today from The Healthy House Institute
430 N. Sewell Road • Bloomington, IN 47408 • 812–332–5073
www.hhinst.com   MasterCard and Visa orders accepted.

Shipping: $3.00 for the first item, plus $2.00 for each additional item.
Overseas shipping: $5.00 for first item, plus $3.00 for each additional item.
Indiana residents add 5% sales tax. Payment must be in U.S. funds.

III THE
HEALTHY HOUSE
INSTITUTE 430 N. Sewell Road   Bloomington, IN 47408   (812) 332–5073

www.hhinst.com

NAME

ADDRESS

CITY, STATE, ZIP

PHONE (   )

DATE

Qty.	Description	Price Each	Amount

PAYMENT METHOD

☐ Check or Money Order   ☐ Master Card   ☐ Visa

Expiration date_____

Signature_____

Subtotal	
Indiana residents add 5% sales tax	
Shipping: $3.00 for the first item and $2.00 for each additional item	
TOTAL	

Shipping for overseas orders: $5.00 for the first item and $3.00 for each additional item. Payment must be in U.S. funds.